Premature Ovarian Failure

A Medical Dictionary, Bibliography,
and Annotated Research Guide to
Internet References

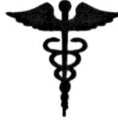

James N. Parker, M.D.
and Philip M. Parker, Ph.D., Editors

ICON Health Publications
ICON Group International, Inc.
4370 La Jolla Village Drive, 4th Floor
San Diego, CA 92122 USA

Copyright ©2004 by ICON Group International, Inc.

Copyright ©2004 by ICON Group International, Inc. All rights reserved. This book is protected by copyright. No part of it may be reproduced, stored in a retrieval system, or transmitted in any form or by any means, electronic, mechanical, photocopying, recording, or otherwise, without written permission from the publisher.

Printed in the United States of America.

Last digit indicates print number: 10 9 8 7 6 4 5 3 2 1

Publisher, Health Care: Philip Parker, Ph.D.
Editor(s): James Parker, M.D., Philip Parker, Ph.D.

Publisher's note: The ideas, procedures, and suggestions contained in this book are not intended for the diagnosis or treatment of a health problem. As new medical or scientific information becomes available from academic and clinical research, recommended treatments and drug therapies may undergo changes. The authors, editors, and publisher have attempted to make the information in this book up to date and accurate in accord with accepted standards at the time of publication. The authors, editors, and publisher are not responsible for errors or omissions or for consequences from application of the book, and make no warranty, expressed or implied, in regard to the contents of this book. Any practice described in this book should be applied by the reader in accordance with professional standards of care used in regard to the unique circumstances that may apply in each situation. The reader is advised to always check product information (package inserts) for changes and new information regarding dosage and contraindications before prescribing any drug or pharmacological product. Caution is especially urged when using new or infrequently ordered drugs, herbal remedies, vitamins and supplements, alternative therapies, complementary therapies and medicines, and integrative medical treatments.

Cataloging-in-Publication Data

Parker, James N., 1961-
Parker, Philip M., 1960-

Premature Ovarian Failure: A Medical Dictionary, Bibliography, and Annotated Research Guide to Internet References / James N. Parker and Philip M. Parker, editors
        p.   cm.
Includes bibliographical references, glossary, and index.
ISBN: 0-497-00906-4
1. Premature Ovarian Failure-Popular works.   I. Title.

Disclaimer

This publication is not intended to be used for the diagnosis or treatment of a health problem. It is sold with the understanding that the publisher, editors, and authors are not engaging in the rendering of medical, psychological, financial, legal, or other professional services.

References to any entity, product, service, or source of information that may be contained in this publication should not be considered an endorsement, either direct or implied, by the publisher, editors, or authors. ICON Group International, Inc., the editors, and the authors are not responsible for the content of any Web pages or publications referenced in this publication.

Copyright Notice

If a physician wishes to copy limited passages from this book for patient use, this right is automatically granted without written permission from ICON Group International, Inc. (ICON Group). However, all of ICON Group publications have copyrights. With exception to the above, copying our publications in whole or in part, for whatever reason, is a violation of copyright laws and can lead to penalties and fines. Should you want to copy tables, graphs, or other materials, please contact us to request permission (E-mail: iconedit@san.rr.com). ICON Group often grants permission for very limited reproduction of our publications for internal use, press releases, and academic research. Such reproduction requires confirmed permission from ICON Group International, Inc. **The disclaimer above must accompany all reproductions, in whole or in part, of this book.**

Acknowledgements

The collective knowledge generated from academic and applied research summarized in various references has been critical in the creation of this book which is best viewed as a comprehensive compilation and collection of information prepared by various official agencies which produce publications on premature ovarian failure. Books in this series draw from various agencies and institutions associated with the United States Department of Health and Human Services, and in particular, the Office of the Secretary of Health and Human Services (OS), the Administration for Children and Families (ACF), the Administration on Aging (AOA), the Agency for Healthcare Research and Quality (AHRQ), the Agency for Toxic Substances and Disease Registry (ATSDR), the Centers for Disease Control and Prevention (CDC), the Food and Drug Administration (FDA), the Healthcare Financing Administration (HCFA), the Health Resources and Services Administration (HRSA), the Indian Health Service (IHS), the institutions of the National Institutes of Health (NIH), the Program Support Center (PSC), and the Substance Abuse and Mental Health Services Administration (SAMHSA). In addition to these sources, information gathered from the National Library of Medicine, the United States Patent Office, the European Union, and their related organizations has been invaluable in the creation of this book. Some of the work represented was financially supported by the Research and Development Committee at INSEAD. This support is gratefully acknowledged. Finally, special thanks are owed to Tiffany Freeman for her excellent editorial support.

About the Editors

James N. Parker, M.D.

Dr. James N. Parker received his Bachelor of Science degree in Psychobiology from the University of California, Riverside and his M.D. from the University of California, San Diego. In addition to authoring numerous research publications, he has lectured at various academic institutions. Dr. Parker is the medical editor for health books by ICON Health Publications.

Philip M. Parker, Ph.D.

Philip M. Parker is the Eli Lilly Chair Professor of Innovation, Business and Society at INSEAD (Fontainebleau, France and Singapore). Dr. Parker has also been Professor at the University of California, San Diego and has taught courses at Harvard University, the Hong Kong University of Science and Technology, the Massachusetts Institute of Technology, Stanford University, and UCLA. Dr. Parker is the associate editor for ICON Health Publications.

About ICON Health Publications

To discover more about ICON Health Publications, simply check with your preferred online booksellers, including Barnes&Noble.com and Amazon.com which currently carry all of our titles. Or, feel free to contact us directly for bulk purchases or institutional discounts:

> ICON Group International, Inc.
> 4370 La Jolla Village Drive, Fourth Floor
> San Diego, CA 92122 USA
> Fax: 858-546-4341
> Web site: **www.icongrouponline.com/health**

Table of Contents

FORWARD	1
CHAPTER 1. STUDIES ON PREMATURE OVARIAN FAILURE	3
Overview	3
Federally Funded Research on Premature Ovarian Failure	3
The National Library of Medicine: PubMed	16
CHAPTER 2. ALTERNATIVE MEDICINE AND PREMATURE OVARIAN FAILURE	61
Overview	61
National Center for Complementary and Alternative Medicine	61
Additional Web Resources	64
General References	65
CHAPTER 3. PATENTS ON PREMATURE OVARIAN FAILURE	67
Overview	67
Patents on Premature Ovarian Failure	67
Patent Applications on Premature Ovarian Failure	69
Keeping Current	70
CHAPTER 4. BOOKS ON PREMATURE OVARIAN FAILURE	71
Overview	71
Book Summaries: Online Booksellers	71
APPENDIX A. PHYSICIAN RESOURCES	75
Overview	75
NIH Guidelines	75
NIH Databases	77
Other Commercial Databases	79
APPENDIX B. PATIENT RESOURCES	81
Overview	81
Patient Guideline Sources	81
Finding Associations	84
APPENDIX C. FINDING MEDICAL LIBRARIES	87
Overview	87
Preparation	87
Finding a Local Medical Library	87
Medical Libraries in the U.S. and Canada	87
ONLINE GLOSSARIES	93
Online Dictionary Directories	93
PREMATURE OVARIAN FAILURE DICTIONARY	95
INDEX	129

FORWARD

In March 2001, the National Institutes of Health issued the following warning: "The number of Web sites offering health-related resources grows every day. Many sites provide valuable information, while others may have information that is unreliable or misleading."[1] Furthermore, because of the rapid increase in Internet-based information, many hours can be wasted searching, selecting, and printing. Since only the smallest fraction of information dealing with premature ovarian failure is indexed in search engines, such as **www.google.com** or others, a non-systematic approach to Internet research can be not only time consuming, but also incomplete. This book was created for medical professionals, students, and members of the general public who want to know as much as possible about premature ovarian failure, using the most advanced research tools available and spending the least amount of time doing so.

In addition to offering a structured and comprehensive bibliography, the pages that follow will tell you where and how to find reliable information covering virtually all topics related to premature ovarian failure, from the essentials to the most advanced areas of research. Public, academic, government, and peer-reviewed research studies are emphasized. Various abstracts are reproduced to give you some of the latest official information available to date on premature ovarian failure. Abundant guidance is given on how to obtain free-of-charge primary research results via the Internet. **While this book focuses on the field of medicine, when some sources provide access to non-medical information relating to premature ovarian failure, these are noted in the text.**

E-book and electronic versions of this book are fully interactive with each of the Internet sites mentioned (clicking on a hyperlink automatically opens your browser to the site indicated). If you are using the hard copy version of this book, you can access a cited Web site by typing the provided Web address directly into your Internet browser. You may find it useful to refer to synonyms or related terms when accessing these Internet databases. **NOTE:** At the time of publication, the Web addresses were functional. However, some links may fail due to URL address changes, which is a common occurrence on the Internet.

For readers unfamiliar with the Internet, detailed instructions are offered on how to access electronic resources. For readers unfamiliar with medical terminology, a comprehensive glossary is provided. For readers without access to Internet resources, a directory of medical libraries, that have or can locate references cited here, is given. We hope these resources will prove useful to the widest possible audience seeking information on premature ovarian failure.

The Editors

---

[1] From the NIH, National Cancer Institute (NCI): **http://www.cancer.gov/cancerinfo/ten-things-to-know**.

CHAPTER 1. STUDIES ON PREMATURE OVARIAN FAILURE

Overview

In this chapter, we will show you how to locate peer-reviewed references and studies on premature ovarian failure.

Federally Funded Research on Premature Ovarian Failure

The U.S. Government supports a variety of research studies relating to premature ovarian failure. These studies are tracked by the Office of Extramural Research at the National Institutes of Health.[2] CRISP (Computerized Retrieval of Information on Scientific Projects) is a searchable database of federally funded biomedical research projects conducted at universities, hospitals, and other institutions.

Search the CRISP Web site at **http://crisp.cit.nih.gov/crisp/crisp_query.generate_screen**. You will have the option to perform targeted searches by various criteria, including geography, date, and topics related to premature ovarian failure.

For most of the studies, the agencies reporting into CRISP provide summaries or abstracts. As opposed to clinical trial research using patients, many federally funded studies use animals or simulated models to explore premature ovarian failure. The following is typical of the type of information found when searching the CRISP database for premature ovarian failure:

- **Project Title: BAYLOR FRAGILE X RESEARCH CENTER**

    Principal Investigator & Institution: Zoghbi, Huda Y.; Professor; Molecular and Human Genetics; Baylor College of Medicine 1 Baylor Plaza Houston, Tx 77030

    Timing: Fiscal Year 2003; Project Start 01-AUG-1988; Project End 30-JUN-2004

---

[2] Healthcare projects are funded by the National Institutes of Health (NIH), Substance Abuse and Mental Health Services (SAMHSA), Health Resources and Services Administration (HRSA), Food and Drug Administration (FDA), Centers for Disease Control and Prevention (CDCP), Agency for Healthcare Research and Quality (AHRQ), and Office of Assistant Secretary of Health (OASH).

Summary: (provided by applicant): This application for supplementary funding to the Baylor College of Medicine Mental Retardation Research Center seeks to establish a collaborative Fragile X Syndrome Research Center composed of investigators at Baylor College of Medicine in Houston, Texas and Emory University School of Medicine in Atlanta, Georgia. The application seeks funding for four investigator-initiated research projects and two core facilities. The four projects will revolve around a common theme of delineating the full spectrum of phenotypes and their underlying bases in humans and mice with genetic alterations in the FMR1 gene. This will include a series of investigations into the consequences of moderately expanded CGG repeats (premutations) that have been linked to **premature ovarian failure** and a late onset neurodegeneration. An Administrative Core will be proposed to facilitate interactions among the four research laboratories and the two institutions, and funding is sought to expand core services currently provided by the Baylor College of Medicine MRRC Mouse Neurobehavior and Synaptic Plasticity Core directed by Drs. Richard Paylor and David Sweatt. Additional funding will allow the core to expand services and to characterize the increased numbers of models anticipated to be created in the proposed Center. The four principal investigators proposing projects are Drs. David Nelson and Richard Paylor of Baylor College of Medicine, and Drs. Stephen Warren and Stephanie Sherman of Emory University. Each of these investigators has developed a strong track record of research into fragile X syndrome, and the group is now in a unique position to investigate this novel pathogenic component of fragile X syndrome. Dr. Sherman will investigate the epidemiology of the human male premutation phenotype that involves late onset tremor and cognitive decline. Dr. Nelson will develop mouse models to study effects of premutations and FMR1 gene overexpression. Dr. Warren will investigate proteins that bind selectively to expanded CGG and which may be important to premutation disease as well as fragile X syndrome, and Dr. Paylor will focus on improved methods for characterizing mouse models of fragile X syndrome and their response to treatment.

Website: http://crisp.cit.nih.gov/crisp/Crisp_Query.Generate_Screen

- **Project Title: CELL-SPECIFIC EXPRESSION IN THE PITUITARY GLAND**

Principal Investigator & Institution: Camper, Sally A.; Professor; Human Genetics; University of Michigan at Ann Arbor 3003 South State, Room 1040 Ann Arbor, Mi 481091274

Timing: Fiscal Year 2004; Project Start 15-JUL-1999; Project End 31-MAY-2009

Summary: (provided by applicant): The pituitary gland contains five different cell types that are specialized in hormone production. Understanding the mechanism of cell specification is important because many body functions depend on it. Genetically engineered mice have proven the roles of several transcription factors and signaling molecules, and the correspondence with human pituitary disease is outstanding. We proved that the homeodomain transcription factor PITX2 has a dosage dependent role in development of the pituitary primordium and in activation of lineage specific transcription factor genes. In humans, PITX2 mutations are a cause of Rieger syndrome and isolated growth hormone deficiency. We propose to test the role of PITX2 in maintenance of differentiated functions of specialized pituitary cells by cell specific deletion in mice. The role of GATA2, a downstream target of PITX2, will be tested using a conditional null allele of Gata2. FOXL2 is a forkhead transcription factor that is one of the earliest markers of differentiated cells in the developing pituitary gland, and it activates gonadotropin releasing hormone receptor transcription. Humans haploinsufficient for FOXL2 have eye defects and **premature ovarian failure**. We propose that FoxI2 has roles in regulating the growth of committed anterior pituitary cells during development, in the function of mature gonadotropes, and in susceptibility to pituitary tumors. We will explore these ideas by characterizing FoxI2 expression, placing it in the genetic hierarchy of known transcription factors, and analyzing the consequences of an inducible loss of function allele in mice. Our understanding of pituitary cell specification would be advanced if we had markers to identify specialized cells prior to terminal differentiation and activation of hormone gene transcription. To generate such markers we propose to compare the transcriptomes of pituitary cell types using transgenic technology to mark cells for purification and gene array analysis. Transcripts unique to each differentiated cell type will be identified by bioinformatics and verified experimentally. During the proposed grant cycle we will have defined the roles of three pituitary transcription factors using well-established methods and initiated a new approach to studying cell specification. We expect that these studies will provide valuable insight for understanding the etiology of human pituitary hormone deficiency diseases and characterization of pituitary adenomas.

Website: http://crisp.cit.nih.gov/crisp/Crisp_Query.Generate_Screen

- **Project Title: CHARACTERIZATION OF THE FRAGILE X MUTATION**

Principal Investigator & Institution: Sherman, Stephanie L.; Professor of Human Genetics; Emory University 1784 North Decatur Road Atlanta, Ga 30322

Timing: Fiscal Year 2002; Project Start 01-JUL-2002; Project End 30-JUN-2003

Summary: The fragile X syndrome (FXS), a type of inherited mental retardation (MR), is due to the silencing of the FMR1 X-linked gene. In over 98% of cases, the mutation is due to an expansion of an unstable CGG repeat sequence located in the 5? untranslated region of the gene. Once over 200 repeats (full mutations), the FMR1 gene is hypermethylated and consequently no message is transcribed. Originally, no significant phenotype was thought to be associated with the 6% of individuals in the general population who carry long, unmethylated FMR1 repeat tracks, i.e., those alleles with 41-199 repeats that produce FMR1 mRNA and protein (FMRP). However, there is now convincing evidence for an associated phenotype: 21% of women who carry the premutation allele (6 1-199 repeats) are at risk for **premature ovarian failure** (POF) while those who carry full mutations have the same risk as the general population. Moreover, preliminary evidence from males indicates that increased levels of FMR1 mRNA and reduced levels of FMRP are associated with increasing repeat number. Based on the applicant?s previous work and that of others, she has suggested that an increased number of FMR1 repeats may influence an individual?s cognitive and behavioral performance. Given the FMR1 gene is known to play a role in normal brain function, examination of a cognitive and behavioral consequence of FMR1 high repeat alleles is an important next step. The applicant proposes to determine the FMR1 mRNA and FMRP levels of high repeat carriers to better define the affect of long CGG repeat tracts and associated phenotypes. Specifically, she plans to assess 650 individuals, including high repeat carriers and controls, on whom she has neuropsychological profiles. In addition, she plans to confirm or refute a recent report suggesting that premutation males may be at risk for late onset cerebellar tremors. Lastly, she thinks it is imperative to begin to translate this important genetic information on the FXS, the most common inherited form of MR, into the public health arena. Because women who carry the premutation are not only at risk for having a child with the FXS but also are at risk for POF, she plans to investigate the feasibility of screening women of reproductive age for premutation alleles. This proposal will take the first step to rigorously assess the consequence of high repeat alleles at the molecular and phenotypic level and then determine if these data can be applied at the public health level.

Website: http://crisp.cit.nih.gov/crisp/Crisp_Query.Generate_Screen

- **Project Title: CONSTITUTIVELY ACTIVE LH RECEPTORS IN TRANSGENIC MICE**

  Principal Investigator & Institution: Narayan, Prema; Biochem and Molecular Biology; University of Georgia 617 Boyd, Gsrc Athens, Ga 306027411

  Timing: Fiscal Year 2004; Project Start 01-JAN-2004; Project End 30-DEC-2007

  Summary: (provided by applicant): The long-term goals of this research are to understand the reproductive consequences of expression of constitutively active luteinizing hormone receptors (LHR). The critical role of LHR in male and female reproduction is underscored by the developmental and reproductive defects resulting from activating and inactivating mutations in the receptor. For example, activating mutations in human LHR are associated with familial male-limited precocious puberty (FMPP) and Leydig cell hyperplasia. Transgenic and knockout mouse models have facilitated our understanding of normal and pathophysiological functions of hormones and receptors. To examine the consequences of chronic ligand-mediated LHR activity, we have generated transgenic mice expressing a yoked hormone-receptor fusion protein (YHR) with constitutive activity. Male transgenic mice produce increased prepubertal levels of testosterone, accompanied by decreased testicular size and diameter of the seminiferous tubules. Female transgenic mice exhibit increased folliculogenesis at early ages, and at three months there is increased follicular atresia and the presence of follicular cysts suggesting that constitutive LHR activity may result in **premature ovarian failure.** The goals of this proposal are to elucidate the endocrine and molecular basis for altered testicular development and early reproductive senescence observed in the ovary. In the first aim we will examine the developmental changes in testicular and ovarian morphology and histology and determine the effect of chronic LHR activation on testicular somatic cell development and oocyte depletion. In the second aim we will analyze the temporal changes in hormone levels and expression of key molecules in the LHR signaling pathways to determine the endocrine and molecular basis of the testicular and ovarian phenotype. These studies will contribute new information on testicular and ovarian physiology and pathophysiology and provide insight into the molecular mechanisms of FMPP, female infertility and **premature ovarian failure.**

  Website: http://crisp.cit.nih.gov/crisp/Crisp_Query.Generate_Screen

- **Project Title: ENVIRONMENTAL EPOXIDES--MECHANISMS OF OVOTOXICITY**

  Principal Investigator & Institution: Hoyer, Patricia B.; Professor; Physiology; University of Arizona P O Box 3308 Tucson, Az 857223308

  Timing: Fiscal Year 2002; Project Start 01-FEB-1999; Project End 31-JAN-2004

  Summary: The environmental chemical, 4-Vinylcyclohexene (VCH) is produced in the manufacture of rubber tires, flame retardants, insecticides, plasticizers, and antioxidants. Dosing (30 d) with the diepoxide metabolite, 4- vinylcyclohexene diepoxide (VCD) destroys the majority of small pre-antral (primordial) follicles in the ovaries of mice and rats. Females are born with a finite number of primordial follicles that cannot be regenerated; thus, chemicals that destroy oocytes contained in these follicles can produce **premature ovarian failure.** Exposure of women to known ovotoxicants such as cigarette smoke and chemotherapeutic agents has been associated with early menopause, thus, potential exposure to other ovotoxic chemicals in the industrial setting is of concern. Previous studies with VCD (80mg/kg) in rats showed that destruction of small follicles requires daily dosing (10 days), is via physiological cell death (apoptosis), and is accompanied by altered expression of genes associated with apoptosis (bax), oxidative stress (superoxide dismutase, and detoxification (epoxide hydrolase). The studies, proposed here will characterize the role of oxidative stress and follicular metabolism in VCD-induced apoptosis. The experimental approach will involve exploiting the shift in responsiveness to VCD dosing we have observed in small follicles from a protective effect (1 dose), to an apoptotic effect (10 and 15 daily doses). Additionally, these studies will use the isolated small follicle system we have developed in conjunction with confocal microscopy to localize events within specific cells. The hypothesis to be tested is that: VCD initiates an oxidative stress response in small preantral follicles that is altered after repeated dosing to trigger the onset of bax- mediated apoptosis. The Specific Aims are 1) to characterize the oxidative stress response in bax-mediated apoptosis, 2) to relate VCD metabolism with oxidative stress in small follicles, and 3) to evaluate the stress-activated pathway to apoptosis. The studies will use an integrated morphological, biochemical and molecular approach to provide a greater understanding of the mechanisms of ovotoxicity caused by occupational, epoxides. The results of these studies will provide greater insight as to the impact of exposure to ovotoxic environmental chemicals on reproductive health in women.

Website: http://crisp.cit.nih.gov/crisp/Crisp_Query.Generate_Screen

- **Project Title: ESTROGEN IN THE ESTABLISHMENT OF PEAK BONE MASS**

Principal Investigator & Institution: Mulder, Jean E.; Medicine; Columbia University Health Sciences Po Box 49 New York, Ny 10032

Timing: Fiscal Year 2002; Project Start 15-SEP-1999; Project End 30-JUN-2004

Summary: Advances in the treatment of childhood cancers have resulted in markedly improved survival rates for many patients. These advancements in therapy, however, have led to new problems, namely, long-term consequences of effective tretments such as the premature loss of gonadal function. **Premature ovarian failure** (POF) places women at great risk for osteoporosis. The issues raised in this research project, however, differ from usual considerations of age-related menopausal ovarian failure and the accelerated bone loss that ensues. This more typical clinical event follows well after the establishment of peak bone mass. The young women to be investigated in this research project have become estrogen deficient before achieving peak bone mass in this setting. The skeletal profile of young women cancer survivors with ovarian failure will be characterized first. Other potential contributing factors, such as androgen deficiency, growth hormone deficiency, chemotherapeutic agents, nutritional, and other metabolic parameters will be evaluated. The dosage of estrogen required to establish peak bone mass optimally will then be determined. In this prospective, longitudinal study, young cancer survivors with POF will be randomized to one of two estrogen replacement regimens (high dose versus conventional dose). Patients will be monitored every three months for 2 years. Evaluations will include peripheral and central measurements of bone density, indices of bone turnover, and endocrine studies. We anticipate that these studies will yield new information regarding the sufficiency of estrogen replacement therapy in establishing peak bone density in young amenorrheic women. My goal is to become an independent investigator in the field of metabolic bone disease. This award will enable me to obtain new skills in clinical research methods, as well as a greater understanding of the relationship between estrogen and bone modeling in young women. The proposal is particularly fitting for a research career award because it sets the groundwork for future studies, which are essential to my development as an independent investigator. My environment is ideally suited for achieving my goals. My sponsor, Dr. Bilezikian, is an internationally recognized investigator in the field of metabolic bone disease and is committed to providing me with the support I need to pursue my research plans as I make my transition to independent investigator. Through my collaboration with Dr. Sklar, I have access to a large number of young female cancer survivors with ovarian failure. Our Metabolic Bone Unit, with its distinguished tradition in metabolic bone research and education, is an excellent environment in which to develop my career as a clinical investigator.

Website: http://crisp.cit.nih.gov/crisp/Crisp_Query.Generate_Screen

- **Project Title: FUNCTIONAL ANALYSIS OF ACTIVINS DURING DEVELOPMENT**

    Principal Investigator & Institution: Matzuk, Martin; Professor; Pathology; Baylor College of Medicine 1 Baylor Plaza Houston, Tx 77030

    Timing: Fiscal Year 2004; Project Start 17-AUG-1994; Project End 30-MAR-2009

    Summary: (provided by applicant): The transforming growth factor beta (TGFbeta) superfamily is the largest family of secreted proteins in mammals. This family includes the activins, inhibins, TGFbetas, bone morphogenetic proteins (BMPs), and growth differentiation factors (GDFs). These ligands signal through an oligomeric complex of transmembrane type I and type II serine/threonine kinase receptors. Ligand-induced heterodimerization of these receptors leads to phosphorylation of receptor-regulated SMAD proteins, which translocate to the nucleus with the common SMAD4 protein and regulate gene expression. The characterization of mice and humans with mutations in these signaling pathways has revealed the diversity of developmental and physiological processes in which this family functions. Through the support of this grant, my laboratory has generated and analyzed mice with mutations in activin subunits, an activin binding protein (follistatin), activin receptor type II, a downstream receptor binding protein (FKBP 12), and SMADS. We have recently shown that mice with granulosa cell ablation of follistatin are a model for **premature ovarian failure** in women. The utility of these knockout mice in defining gene function in vivo is unparalleled, and these powerful genetic models have been indispensable for investigating development and reproduction. The overall hypothesis of this R01 renewal is that we will be able to dissect the TGFbeta signaling pathways in the ovary using available and newly-created ovary-specific knockout mouse models. These studies will allow us to place ligands, receptors, and downstream SMAD proteins into biological pathways in a single cell type (i.e., The granulosa cells of the ovary). The Specific Aims of the proposed studies are as follows: 1) Produce transgenic models to define the intraovarian roles of activins; 2) Dissect the activin receptor type II, BMP receptor type II, and BMP receptor type I signaling pathways in the ovary; and 3) Study the interrelationships of the downstream SMAD proteins in ovarian physiology. Generation and characterization of these transgenic mice will define essential and interacting TGFa superfamily signaling components and pathways in the ovary and will continue to be important models for human reproductive diseases including infertility, **premature ovarian failure,** polycystic ovary syndrome, and ovarian cancer.

    Website: http://crisp.cit.nih.gov/crisp/Crisp_Query.Generate_Screen

- **Project Title: GENETICS OF COGNITION IN ADULT TURNER SYNDROME**

    Principal Investigator & Institution: Ross, Judith L.; Professor; Pediatrics; Thomas Jefferson University Office of Research Administration Philadelphia, Pa 191075587

    Timing: Fiscal Year 2002; Project Start 17-MAY-2001; Project End 30-APR-2006

Summary: (adapted from applicant's abstract): Turner syndrome (TS) is the human genetic disorder involving females who lack all or part of one X chromosome. The complex phenotype includes ovarian failure, a characteristic neurocognitive profile, and typical physical features. TS features are associated not only with complete monosomy X but also with partial deletions of either the short (Xp) or long (Xq) arm (partial monosomy X). Impaired visual-spatial/perceptual abilities are characteristic of TS children and adults of varying races and socioeconomic status, but global developmental delay is uncommon. The constellation of neurocognitive deficits observed in TS is most likely multifactorial and related to a complex interaction between genetic abnormalities, hormonal deficiencies, and other unspecified determinants of cognitive ability. Furthermore, an additional genetic mechanism, imprinting, may contribute to cognitive deficits associated with monosomy X. The investigators propose in the current study to delineate the genetic factors that account for the Turner syndrome neurocognitive phenotype in adults by 1) mapping the TS-associated neurocognitive phenotypes in partial monosomy X women, 2) collecting parent-of-origin data from adult Turner syndrome subjects for imprinting studies, and 3) contrasting women who have both genetic (X chromosome) and hormonal abnormalities with women who have only a hormonal abnormality (idiopathic premature ovarian failure). These studies will test the hypothesis from preliminary data that cognitive dysfunction associated with monosomy X maps to distal Xp. As a relatively common genetic disorder with well-defined manifestations, TS presents an opportunity to investigate genetic factors that influence female cognitive development. There is potentially informative genetic and phenotypic variation among TS subjects with partial X deletions. Careful clinical and molecular characterization of these unusual subjects, who represent "experiments in nature," could link the TS phenotype of impaired visual spatial/perceptual ability to specific X chromosome regions. Turner syndrome is an excellent model for such phenotype mapping studies because of its prevalence, the well-characterized phenotype, and the wealth of molecular resources available for the X chromosome. Phenotype mapping of X deletions will be helpful for genetic counseling. Characterization of specific TS causative genes would provide insight into the pathophysiology of 45,X, Turner syndrome, as well as the process of normal neurocognitive development.

Website: http://crisp.cit.nih.gov/crisp/CrIsp_Query.Generate_Screen

- **Project Title: IGF-I SIGNALING IN GRANULOSA CELLS**

  Principal Investigator & Institution: Davis, John S.; Professor and Director of Research and d; Obstetrics and Gynecology; University of Nebraska Medical Center Omaha, Ne 681987835

  Timing: Fiscal Year 2002; Project Start 01-MAY-2001; Project End 31-JUL-2005

  Summary: (Scanned from the applicant's abstract) The intrafollicular IGF-I system amplifies gonadotropin hormone action in granulosa cells. IGF-I alone or in combination with FSH can induce gonadotropin receptors, steroidogenic enzymes and promote follicular survival. The important interplay among IGF-I and FSH is underscored by the striking similarity of ovaries in IGF-I knockout, FSH knockout and FSH receptor knockout mice. The follicles in these mice are arrested in the early antral stage of development. Whereas the mechanism of action of FSH is well known to involve the cAMP/protein kinase A signaling pathway, almost nothing is known about the intracellular actions of IGF-I in the ovary. Furthermore, recent studies by others and our preliminary data suggest that some of the signaling pathways utilized by IGF-I and FSH converge. The proposed studies are designed to test the overall hypothesis that IGF-I induced Pl-3-kinase signaling pathway is required for granulosa cell survival and amplification of FSH-induced granulosa cell differentiation. The specific questions to be answered in this proposal are: Aim 1) Are the signaling events initiated by IGF-I amplified in response to FSH? Hypothesis: The IGF-I dependent Pl-3-kinase signaling pathway in granulosa cells is augmented by FSH. Aim 2) Are the survival effects of IGF-I and FSH mediated by parallel or converging intracellular signaling pathways? Hypothesis I: The survival effects of IGF-I and FSH are mediated by Pl-3-kinase/Akt mediated phosphorylation of Bad. Hypothesis II: IGF-I and FSH elevate the cellular ratio of antiapoptotic (e.g., Bc12, Bcl-Xlong, Mci-I) to pro -apoptotic proteins (e.g., Bad, Bax, Bok) and inhibit caspase activity. Aim 3) Is FSH directed granulosa cell differentiation mediated via IGF-I dependent signaling systems? Hypothesis: IGF-I stimulated Pl-3-kinase signaling events amplifies FSH directed expression of differentiation, whereas ERK signaling represses djfferentiation. We will employ specific chemical inhibitors and adenovirus vectors that express dominant negative or active signaling molecules to dissect the IGF-I and FSH directed signaling pathways that are responsible for granulosa cell survival or granulosa cell differentiation. Further characterization of the IGF-I and FSH signaling events and their interactions are likely to provide new insights into how multiple genes are coordinately regulated by trophic factors during follicle development. Our studies are expected to translate into more effective treatments for controlling follicle selection and development, ovulation and fertility. This new insight may uncover mechanistic defects that underlay disorders of folliculogenesis, **premature ovarian failure** and disorders such as polycystic ovarian syndrome.

Website: http://crisp.cit.nih.gov/crisp/Crisp_Query.Generate_Screen

- **Project Title: OVARIAN-MIMETIC SCAFFOLDS FOR CULTURE /OVARIAN FOLLICLES**

    Principal Investigator & Institution: Shea, Lonnie D.; Assistant Professor; Northwestern University 633 Clark Street Evanston, Il 602081110

    Timing: Fiscal Year 2003; Project Start 23-APR-2003; Project End 31-MAR-2008

    Summary: Standard in vitro fertilization procedures cannot preserve the reproductive potential of women in all situations, such as **premature ovarian failure** or oncotherapy induced sterility. The in vitro maturation of granulosa cell-oocyte complexes (GOC) may provide an alternative to current methodology. The goal of this project is to employ a three-dimensional, engineered, synthetic stroma to examine GOC maturation and development in vitro. The central hypothesis underlying this proposal is that the development of the granulosa cells and the oocyte must be coordinated to allow effective maturation of the oocyte to provide fertilization. Oocyte maturation and granulosa cell development involve endocrine, paracrine, and autocrine-acting factors in addition to appropriate somatic-germ cell and cell-matrix interactions. The native stroma surrounding a GOC dynamically regulates growth and maturation by maintaining cellular interactions and providing the matrix interactions that direct cell function. We will employ an atginatebased scaffold as a synthetic stroma that provides the factors that stimulate development and removes the factors that inhibit maturation. Alginate exhibits minimal cellular interactions and thus provides an environment that can be designed to present specific stimuli. Preliminary results have demonstrated gentle encapsulation of individual GOCs within beads and that cultured complexes retain their normal architecture. GOCs produce estradiol in response to growth and differentiation factors. Importantly, retrieved oocyte undergo germinal vesicle breakdown and fertilization results in the development to the two-cell stage. We specifically aim to use this system to examine the coordination of GOC development and oocyte maturation by 1) mechanically supporting the GOC to maintain the cell-cell interactions 2) supplying growth and differentiation factors, and 3) regulating the granulosa cell-matrix interactions. We systematically examine the role of each component in directing the cellular processes within the developing GOC, and thereby the ultimate maturation of the oocyte in vitro. This three-dimensional culture system may provide novel therapeutic approaches for germline preservation.

Website: http://crisp.cit.nih.gov/crisp/Crisp_Query.Generate_Screen

- **Project Title: PREMATURE OVARIAN FAILURE IN BREAST CANCER PATIENTS**

    Principal Investigator & Institution: Shapiro, Charles; Brigham and Women's Hospital 75 Francis Street Boston, Ma 02115

    Timing: Fiscal Year 2002

    Summary: The purposes of this research study are to (1) evaluate bone mineral density and bone metabolism in premenopausal women with breast cancer who receive adjuvant chemotherapy and (2) to determine whether nasal spray calcitonin prevents or mitigates short term bone loss in ppremenopausal women with breast cancer.

    Website: http://crisp.cit.nih.gov/crisp/Crisp_Query.Generate_Screen

- **Project Title: PREVENTION OF OSTEOPOROSIS IN BREAST CANCER SURVIVORS**

    Principal Investigator & Institution: Waltman, Nancy L.; Adult Health and Illness; University of Nebraska Medical Center Omaha, Ne 681987835

    Timing: Fiscal Year 2002; Project Start 01-APR-2002; Project End 31-DEC-2006

    Summary: Osteoporosis can be a major debilitating, expensive, long term, irreversible condition, and breast cancer survivors are particularly at risk for osteoporosis. As a result of some chemotherapy agents, many of these women experience **premature ovarian failure.** At least 60% of women with breast cancer have estrogen receptor positive tumor status; thus, they are not candidates for hormone replacement therapy. Without estrogen, bone loss occurs rapidly the first five years of menopause and continues over time but at a slower rate. The purpose of this study is to test whether strength/weight training exercises enhance the effectiveness of risedronate (5 mg/day), calcium (1200 mg/day), and vitamin D (400 IU/day) in improving bone mineral density (BMD) in post-menopausal breast cancer survivors. The sample will be 218 subjects recruited within a 100 mile radius of r sites across Nebraska (Omaha, Lincoln, Kearney and Scottsbluff). Post-menopausal women with a history of stage O (in situ), stage I or II breast cancer, with a BMD DEXA T-score of -1.0 SD or lower at any of 3 sites (hip, spine, forearm) will be stratified by time since menopause (5 yrs or less: > 5 years) and randomly assigned to one of two treatment groups (G1 and G2), with approximately 109 per group. Differences in tamoxifen, smoking, intake of calcium, and body mass index (BMI) between the two groups at baseline will be examined; if differences exist they will be controlled statistically. Both groups will receive risedronate, calcium and vitamin D; G1 also will receive strength/weight training exercises for upper and lower extremities and spine. Facilitative strategies based on Bandura's (1997) Self-Efficacy Theory are designed and used to encourage long-term adherence for both groups. The multi-component intervention is 24 months with follow-up at 30 and 36 months. The primary outcome measure is BMD of the hip, spine and forearm (via DEXA): secondary outcome measures are muscle strength and fractures. The impact of the multi-component intervention on outcomes will be assessed using General Estimating Equation methodology Measurement of outcomes will occur at 6 and/or 12 month intervals through 36 months. In addition, relationships will be examined between level of confidence in goal accomplishment and adherence to intervention components over time. This study may provide evidence of an effective alternative to HRT for treatment of osteoporosis in breast cancer survivors who are not candidates for HRT.

Website: http://crisp.cit.nih.gov/crisp/Crisp_Query.Generate_Screen

- **Project Title: PROTEIN TARGETS OF OVARIAN AND OOCYTE AUTOANTIBODIES**

Principal Investigator & Institution: Luborsky, Judith L.; Rush University Medical Center Chicago, Il 60612

Timing: Fiscal Year 2003; Project Start 01-MAR-2003; Project End 28-FEB-2008

Summary: (provided by applicant): There is compelling evidence for an autoimmune disease of the ovary. Ovarian autoimmunity may affect 1-2 million women in the US. In order to identify women with ovarian autoimmunity we developed prototype immunoassays to detect ovary specific autoantibodies, and used them to develop phenotypic information on the association of ovarian autoimmunity with premature menopause (premature ovarian failure or POF) and unexplained infertility. Further human research and clinical use depends on identification of the relevant protein antigens. The objective of the proposed study is to identify major autoantigens relevant to the phenotypes associated with ovarian autoimmunity. Previous studies suggest that ovary specific autoantibodies react with several ovarian antigens. In addition, autoimmune sera react with four predominant bands of ovarian protein in one-dimensional Western blots. This is consistent with other autoimmune diseases in which antibodies to multiple antigens have the most significant predictive value for disease. We will test the hypothesis that positive sera react with more than one major ovarian antigen (Aim 1). Proteomics methodology combined with the use of a systematically selected panel of autoimmune sera will be used to identify major protein antigens. Recombinant forms of the identified human proteins will be produced. The reaction of each identified protein with the autoimmune sera test panel will be evaluated to verify the authenticity of identified proteins. In Aim 2 the hypothesis that autoimmune POF and unexplained infertility share the same antigens will be tested in order to support the concept that they represent different stages of the same autoimmune disorder. The reaction of sera from women with POF and unexplained infertility will be compared by immunoassay using the identified proteins produced in Aim 1. Furthermore, previous studies showed that ovarian antibodies are associated with a low likelihood of pregnancy after infertility treatment. In Aim 3, the hypothesis that autoantibodies to identified proteins also predict a low likelihood of pregnancy in women with unexplained infertility after in-vitro fertilization will be tested. We will determine if autoantibodies to one antigen or a combination of antigens has predictive value for pregnancy. The proposed study is expected to improve the precision with which ovarian autoimmunity is detected. This will permit studies of disease pathogenesis, health risks associated with ovarian autoimmunity, genetic factors associated with disease susceptibility and improve clinical diagnosis. It will also contribute to a better understanding of an autoimmune disease that affects women's health.

Website: http://crisp.cit.nih.gov/crisp/Crisp_Query.Generate_Screen

- **Project Title: REGULATION OF OOCYTE VIABILITY BY GRANULOSA CELL CONTACT**

    Principal Investigator & Institution: Peluso, John J.; Professor of Physiology and Ob/Gyn; Cell Biology; University of Connecticut Sch of Med/Dnt Bb20, Mc 2806 Farmington, Ct 060302806

    Timing: Fiscal Year 2003; Project Start 01-AUG-2003; Project End 31-JUL-2005

    Summary: (provided by applicant): Menopause occurs once the number of primordial follicles is depleted. Moreover, a rapid depletion of primordial follicles is associated with the age-related decline in fertility and **premature ovarian failure.** It has been estimated that about 70% of these follicles are lost because of oocyte death. Other than this, extremely little is known about the mechanism by which these small follicles are maintained. Insight into the survival mechanisms that influence primordial follicles could come from understanding how these follicles are formed. During embryonic development, primordial germ cells (PGCs) migrate into the developing mammalian ovary, proliferate and then enter meiotic prophase. At this stage, many of the PGCs die via a specific pathway known as apoptosis. However, some PGCs establish contact with somatic cells (presumptive granulosa cells) to form primordial follicles. These PGCs, now referred to as oocytes, appear to be protected from undergoing apoptosis. This process occurs in all mammalian species including humans. While it has been known for decades that cell contact seems to protect oocytes from dying, the mechanism through which cell contact promotes oocyte survival is completely unknown. It is known that granulosa cell-oocyte interaction is mediated, in part, by the adhesion proteins, E- and N-cadherin. Based on our previous studies of granulosa cell apoptosis, we propose that E- and/or N-cadherin mediated cell contact stimulates phosphatidylinositol 3 kinase (PI3K) activity within the oocyte. It is further proposed that PI3K ultimately acts to maintain the viability of the oocyte. Understanding how granulosa cells interact with oocytes to preserve oocyte viability could provide important insights into various aspects of infertility and the mechanisms that control entry into menopause. Therefore, we will determine: 1) the effect of granulosa cell contact on the rate at which oocytes undergo apoptosis in vitro; 2) whether E- and/or N-cadherin mediated cell contact regulates oocyte viability; and 3) whether E- and/or N-cadherin mediated cell contact stimulates PI3K activity and thereby maintains oocyte viability.

    Website: http://crisp.cit.nih.gov/crisp/Crisp_Query.Generate_Screen

- **Project Title: ROLE OF INTEGRINS AND ACTIVIN IN GRANULOSA CELL GROWTH**

    Principal Investigator & Institution: Oktay, Kutluk H.; Obstetrics and Gynecology; Weill Medical College of Cornell Univ New York, Ny 10021

    Timing: Fiscal Year 2003; Project Start 01-FEB-2003; Project End 31-JAN-2008

    Summary: (provided by applicant): The factors that regulate granulosa cell growth during the early stages of follicular development are unknown. Preliminary work showed that extracellular matrix (ECM) plays a role in growth of early stage follicles in concert with activin-A, and suggested an interaction between integrin- and activin/TFG a-signaling pathways. The elucidation of the molecular mechanisms involved in the growth of granulosa cells of early stage follicles may result in the development of therapeutic strategies that prevent **premature ovarian failure,** treat age-related infertility, delay menopause and prevent gonadal damage due to cancer drugs. The applicant focused on the mechanisms behind regulation of early stages of follicle growth since the completion of the clinical training in Reproductive Endocrinology. After a year of research training in the UK with an internationally recognized reproductive biologist, the candidate began studying integrin signaling in ovarian follicle growth in collaboration with the proposed mentor of this project. The applicant's and the mentor's institution is a tri-institutional conglamerate with worldwide recognition in research and top research resources. The mentor is an NIH-funded and world recognized expert in integrin-signaling. The applicant's short-term goals are to strengthen the fund of knowledge in cell and molecular biology, become efficient in techniques to study cell signaling and to generate preliminary data. The candidates' long-term goal is to become an independent clinician-scientist with focus on translating basic research on early follicle growth to clinical applications. To achieve these goals, the applicant proposes a phased development plan where didactic training will be completed during the first three years along with performance of the experiments of Specific Aim-1. The fourth and fifth years will focus on the experiments of second and third aims. The specific aims of this proposal are to investigate and delineate the mechanisms of the interaction between the ECM and activin-A in spontaneously immortalized (SIGC) and primary granulosa cells in parallel, and to determine whether granulosa cell proliferation can be modulated by blockage of this interaction. In pursuit of these specific aims, SIGC will be cultured on polylysine, fibronectin, laminin or collagen in the presence or absence of activin-A. The mechanisms of interaction will be investigated by studying the expression of integrins and activin receptors as well as the expression and phosphorylation of the key integrin and TGFa/activin signaling molecules by Western blotting, in vivo phosphorylation, kinase assays, and immunofluorescence. Expression of transcription factors such as c-jun and c-fos, which are regulated by integrin signaling, will be studied by Western blotting and promoter assays. To pinpoint the mechanism of interaction between the ECM and activin-A, transfection techniques with dominant-negative mutants of the signaling proteins implicated in the interaction between activin-A and the ECM, and specific inhibitors of signaling molecules will be utilized. Cell proliferation and survival will be determined before and after transfection with the dominant-negative mutants.

Website: http://crisp.cit.nih.gov/crisp/Crisp_Query.Generate_Screen

- **Project Title: SEX STEROIDS PROGRAM PREMATURE OVARIAN FAILURE**

    Principal Investigator & Institution: Padmanabhan, Vasantha; Professor of Pediatrics; University of Michigan at Ann Arbor 3003 South State, Room 1040 Ann Arbor, Mi 481091274

    Timing: Fiscal Year 2004; Project Start 01-AUG-2004; Project End 31-JUL-2009

    Summary: Each woman is endowed with a finite number of primordial follicles at birth. Most of this initial endowment is depleted during normal reproductive life, mainly through atresia. The length of reproductive life is largely defined by the rate of follicular depletion. The variability in the length of reproductive life suggests variability in the initial endowment of primordial follicles and/or rate of follicle loss. Reproductive life span can be shortened by factors that reduce primordial follicular endowment, accelerate the rate of recruitment/atresia of follicles, and/or induce follicular deficiencies leading to developmental arrest of follicles. Increasing evidence suggests that the environment to which the fetus is exposed can alter the path of reproductive organ differentiation. The use of animal models offers exciting potential for delineating the mechanisms by which human fertility disorders can be programmed in fetal life. Our studies found that prenatal exposure of sheep to testosterone results in altered neuroendocrine feedback, hyperandrogenism, multifollicular ovarian morphology, increased follicular atresia and reproductive cycle defects culminating in early reproductive failure. The objective of this proposal is to delineate the ovarian programming that occurs as a consequence of in utero sex steroid exposure that is responsible for reproductive failure later in life. The working hypothesis is as follows: Exposure of fetuses to excess testosterone during critical stages of ovarian follicular development alters normal developmental trajectories by changing the expression patterns of key growth factors, androgen/estrogen receptors, and ratio of anti- to proapoptotic Bcl-2 members, resulting in accelerated recruitment of primordial to primary follicles, accelerated growth of primary follicles to antral stage and enhanced incidences of atresia or arrest of antral follicles. These alterations eventually, lead to premature depletion of ovarian follicular reserve and ovarian failure. The deleterious effects of testosterone are mediated either by its androgenic action, estrogenic action due to its conversion to estradiol, or both. Further, prenatal exposure to steroids alters ovarian follicular susceptibility to postnatal steroids leading to **premature ovarian failure.** The outcome of these studies is of relevance to 3 of the targeted NIH missions, fetal antecedents of disease, developmental biology and reproductive health for the 21st century.

Website: http://crisp.cit.nih.gov/crisp/Crisp_Query.Generate_Screen

- **Project Title: TRANSCRIPTIONAL REGULATION OF EARLY FOLLICULOGENESIS**

    Principal Investigator & Institution: Rajkovic, Aleksandar; Molecular and Human Genetics; Baylor College of Medicine 1 Baylor Plaza Houston, Tx 77030

    Timing: Fiscal Year 2004; Project Start 01-APR-2004; Project End 31-MAR-2009

    Summary: (provided by applicant): Oogenesis is a specialized and regulated process essential for ovarian development, embryogenesis and homeostasis. Pathologic changes in both regulatory and structural components of this pathway affect ovarian differentiation, maintenance, and early embryogenesis. A basic understanding of the biologic modifiers important in oogenesis, especially those, which act on the transcriptional level, would further our understanding of oocyte biology as well as provide insight into pathologic processes including **premature ovarian failure,** reproductive life span, menopause, ovarian tumors and early embryonic losses. Identification and characterization of genes preferentially expressed in oocytes will be extremely useful in unraveling their oocyte-specific functions and their contribution to ovarian pathology. We utilized in silico subtraction of expressed sequence tags (ESTs) derived from newborn ovary library to discover a novel homeobox gene preferentially expressed in primordial follicles and growing oocytes, which we call Nobox. Nobox is expressed early in folliculogenesis and may play important roles in regulating mammalian oogenesis. To further study the role of Nobox in ovarian development we generated mice homozygous for the Nobox mutant allele using gene targeting by homologous recombination. Ovaries from mice deficient in Nobox can form primordial follicles but fail to grow and by 6 weeks of age are small and lack discernable follicles and oocytes. The histology of these ovaries closely resembles ovaries from women with afollicular type of non-syndromic **premature ovarian failure.** We propose to study cellular and molecular mechanisms that block follicular development and cause accelerated loss of oocytes in Nobox -/- ovaries. We will characterize NOBOX DNA binding sites and identify genes regulated directly and indirectly by Nobox. We also propose to identify and analyze proteins that interact with NOBOX. These studies will help add to the rapidly increasing amount of information delineating oocyte-specific genetic pathways and to our understanding of the pathologic consequences of mutations in the genes that encode them.

Website: http://crisp.cit.nih.gov/crisp/Crisp_Query.Generate_Screen

- **Project Title: WATER MOVEMENT DURING CELL DEATH**

  Principal Investigator & Institution: Hughes, Francis M.; Biology; University of North Carolina Charlotte Office of Research Services Charlotte, Nc 282230001

  Timing: Fiscal Year 2002; Project Start 09-MAR-2001; Project End 28-FEB-2004

  Summary: Apoptosis is a genetically programmed process of cell death that has recently been implicated in a number of important diseases including a variety of reproductive disorders. In mammals, greater than 99.9% of all oocytes are lost in a process termed atresia which is characterized by massive apoptosis of the supporting granulosa cells. Morphologically, one of the earliest conserved events of dying cells is cell shrinkage and recent studies by the principle investigator and others have identified and rapid and specific efflux of intracellular K+ thought to drive this change. In these studies, K+ efflux caused cell shrinkage by osmotically drawing water out of the dying cell and it was assumed that this water would leave by simple diffusion through the lipid bilayer. In this proposal we challenge that assumption and hypothesize that water movement during apoptosis is mediated by preliminary data that general inhibitors of aquaporins block granulosa cell shrinkage during apoptosis. In addition, these inhibitors also block DNA degradation, leading us to further hypothesize that aquaporin-mediated water loss is critical to down-stream apoptotic events. PCR studies demonstrate that aquaporin-8 and -9 mRNA are expressed in granulosa cells and preliminary antisense studies point to a major role for aquaporin-9 in both cell shrinkage and DNA degradation during cell death. We thus propose a series of studies to assess the role of aquaporins in mediating wa6ter movement and their importance to the overall apoptotic process. These studies will provide the critical pool-of-concept data necessary to submit an R01 application. Defects in aquaporins have been casually implicated in a number of important ailments such as congestive heart failure, pulmonary obstruction cystic fibrosis cataracts asthma and stroke. Thus, it seems likely that alterations in their function may underlie some of the serious diseases associated with apoptosis such a cancer and AIDS as well as those which adversely effect women's health such as **premature ovarian failure,** ovarian cyst formation and ovarian cancer.

  Website: http://crisp.cit.nih.gov/crisp/Crisp_Query.Generate_Screen

The National Library of Medicine: PubMed

One of the quickest and most comprehensive ways to find academic studies in both English and other languages is to use PubMed, maintained by the National Library of Medicine.[3] The advantage of PubMed over previously mentioned sources is that it covers a greater number of domestic and foreign references. It is also free to use. If the publisher has a Web site that offers full text of its journals, PubMed will provide links to that site, as well as to sites offering other related data. User registration, a subscription fee, or some other type of fee may be required to access the full text of articles in some journals.

---

[3] PubMed was developed by the National Center for Biotechnology Information (NCBI) at the National Library of Medicine (NLM) at the National Institutes of Health (NIH). The PubMed database was developed in conjunction with publishers of biomedical literature as a search tool for accessing literature citations and linking to full-text journal articles at Web sites of participating publishers. Publishers that participate in PubMed supply NLM with their citations electronically prior to or at the time of publication.

To generate your own bibliography of studies dealing with premature ovarian failure, simply go to the PubMed Web site at http://www.ncbi.nlm.nih.gov/pubmed. Type "premature ovarian failure" (or synonyms) into the search box, and click "Go." The following is the type of output you can expect from PubMed for premature ovarian failure (hyperlinks lead to article summaries):

- **3 beta hydroxysteroid dehydrogenase autoantibodies in patients with idiopathic premature ovarian failure target N- and C-terminal epitopes.**
  Author(s): Arif S, Varela-Calvino R, Conway GS, Peakman M.
  Source: The Journal of Clinical Endocrinology and Metabolism. 2001 December; 86(12): 5892-7.
  http://www.ncbi.nlm.nih.gov/entrez/query.fcgi?cmd=Retrieve&db=pubmed&dopt=Abstract&list_uids=11739460

- **3beta-hydroxysteroid dehydrogenase autoantibodies are rare in premature ovarian failure.**
  Author(s): Reimand K, Peterson P, Hyoty H, Uibo R, Cooke I, Weetman AP, Krohn KJ.
  Source: The Journal of Clinical Endocrinology and Metabolism. 2000 June; 85(6): 2324-6.
  http://www.ncbi.nlm.nih.gov/entrez/query.fcgi?cmd=Retrieve&db=pubmed&dopt=Abstract&list_uids=10852471

- **45,X/46,XX mosaicism in patients with idiopathic premature ovarian failure.**
  Author(s): Devi AS, Metzger DA, Luciano AA, Benn PA.
  Source: Fertility and Sterility. 1998 July; 70(1): 89-93.
  http://www.ncbi.nlm.nih.gov/entrez/query.fcgi?cmd=Retrieve&db=pubmed&dopt=Abstract&list_uids=9660427

- **47,XXX in an adolescent with premature ovarian failure and autoimmune disease.**
  Author(s): Holland CM.
  Source: Journal of Pediatric and Adolescent Gynecology. 2001 May; 14(2): 77-80.
  http://www.ncbi.nlm.nih.gov/entrez/query.fcgi?cmd=Retrieve&db=pubmed&dopt=Abstract&list_uids=11479104

- **A case of Gitelman's syndrome with premature ovarian failure.**
  Author(s): Akalin A, Kasifoglu T, Efe B.
  Source: Clinical Nephrology. 2002 July; 58(1): 81-2.
  http://www.ncbi.nlm.nih.gov/entrez/query.fcgi?cmd=Retrieve&db=pubmed&dopt=Abstract&list_uids=12141414

- **A combination of gonadotropin-releasing hormone analog and human menopausal gonadotropins for ovulation induction in premature ovarian failure.**
  Author(s): Letterie G, Miyazawa K.
  Source: Acta Obstetricia Et Gynecologica Scandinavica. 1989; 68(6): 571-3.
  http://www.ncbi.nlm.nih.gov/entrez/query.fcgi?cmd=Retrieve&db=pubmed&dopt=Abstract&list_uids=2520819

- **A controlled study of danazol for the treatment of karyotypically normal spontaneous premature ovarian failure.**
  Author(s): Anasti JN, Kimzey LM, Defensor RA, White B, Nelson LM.
  Source: Fertility and Sterility. 1994 October; 62(4): 726-30.
  http://www.ncbi.nlm.nih.gov/entrez/query.fcgi?cmd=Retrieve&db=pubmed&dopt=Abstract&list_uids=7926080

- **A familial case of X chromosome deletion ascertained by cytogenetic screening of women with premature ovarian failure.**
  Author(s): Davison RM, Quilter CR, Webb J, Murray A, Fisher AM, Valentine A, Serhal P, Conway GS.
  Source: Human Reproduction (Oxford, England). 1998 November; 13(11): 3039-41.
  http://www.ncbi.nlm.nih.gov/entrez/query.fcgi?cmd=Retrieve&db=pubmed&dopt=Abstract&list_uids=9853851

- **A gene for premature ovarian failure associated with eyelid malformation maps to chromosome 3q22-q23.**
  Author(s): Amati P, Gasparini P, Zlotogora J, Zelante L, Chomel JC, Kitzis A, Kaplan J, Bonneau D.
  Source: American Journal of Human Genetics. 1996 May; 58(5): 1089-92.
  http://www.ncbi.nlm.nih.gov/entrez/query.fcgi?cmd=Retrieve&db=pubmed&dopt=Abstract&list_uids=8651270

- **A genetic explanation for premature ovarian failure?**
  Author(s): Senior K.
  Source: Lancet. 2001 February 3; 357(9253): 367.
  http://www.ncbi.nlm.nih.gov/entrez/query.fcgi?cmd=Retrieve&db=pubmed&dopt=Abstract&list_uids=11211007

- **A human homologue of the Drosophila melanogaster diaphanous gene is disrupted in a patient with premature ovarian failure: evidence for conserved function in oogenesis and implications for human sterility.**
  Author(s): Bione S, Sala C, Manzini C, Arrigo G, Zuffardi O, Banfi S, Borsani G, Jonveaux P, Philippe C, Zuccotti M, Ballabio A, Toniolo D.
  Source: American Journal of Human Genetics. 1998 March; 62(3): 533-41.
  http://www.ncbi.nlm.nih.gov/entrez/query.fcgi?cmd=Retrieve&db=pubmed&dopt=Abstract&list_uids=9497258

- **A morphometric study of the uterine glandular epithelium in women with premature ovarian failure undergoing hormone replacement therapy.**
  Author(s): Dockery P, Tidey RR, Li TC, Cooke ID.
  Source: Human Reproduction (Oxford, England). 1991 November; 6(10): 1354-64.
  http://www.ncbi.nlm.nih.gov/entrez/query.fcgi?cmd=Retrieve&db=pubmed&dopt=Abstract&list_uids=1770126

- **A mouse gene encoding an oocyte antigen associated with autoimmune premature ovarian failure.**
  Author(s): Tong ZB, Nelson LM.
  Source: Endocrinology. 1999 August; 140(8): 3720-6.
  http://www.ncbi.nlm.nih.gov/entrez/query.fcgi?cmd=Retrieve&db=pubmed&dopt=Abstract&list_uids=10433232

- **A proportion of patients with premature ovarian failure show lowered percentages of blood monocyte derived dendritic cells capable of forming clusters with lymphocytes.**
  Author(s): Hoek A, van Kasteren Y, de Haan-Meulman M, Schoemaker J, Drexhage HA.
  Source: Advances in Experimental Medicine and Biology. 1993; 329: 629-32.
  http://www.ncbi.nlm.nih.gov/entrez/query.fcgi?cmd=Retrieve&db=pubmed&dopt=Abstract&list_uids=8379437

- **A search for antibodies to luteinizing hormone receptors in premature ovarian failure.**
  Author(s): Austin GE, Coulam CB, Ryan RJ.
  Source: Mayo Clinic Proceedings. 1979 June; 54(6): 394-400.
  http://www.ncbi.nlm.nih.gov/entrez/query.fcgi?cmd=Retrieve&db=pubmed&dopt=Abstract&list_uids=221753

- **A search for immunoglobulins inhibiting gonadal cell steroidogenesis in premature ovarian failure.**
  Author(s): Lambert A, Weetman AP, McLoughlin J, Wardle C, Sunderland J, Wheatcroft N, Anobile C, Robertson WR.
  Source: Human Reproduction (Oxford, England). 1996 September; 11(9): 1871-6.
  http://www.ncbi.nlm.nih.gov/entrez/query.fcgi?cmd=Retrieve&db=pubmed&dopt=Abstract&list_uids=8921056

- **A study of premature ovarian failure in Turkish women.**
  Author(s): Gokmen O, Seckin NC, Sener AB, Ozaksit G, Ekmekci S.
  Source: Gynecological Endocrinology : the Official Journal of the International Society of Gynecological Endocrinology. 1995 December; 9(4): 283-7.
  http://www.ncbi.nlm.nih.gov/entrez/query.fcgi?cmd=Retrieve&db=pubmed&dopt=Abstract&list_uids=8629455

- **Absence of mutations in the coding regions of follicle-stimulating hormone receptor gene in Singapore Chinese women with premature ovarian failure and polycystic ovary syndrome.**
  Author(s): Tong Y, Liao WX, Roy AC, Ng SC.
  Source: Hormone and Metabolic Research. Hormon- Und Stoffwechselforschung. Hormones Et Metabolisme. 2001 April; 33(4): 221-6.
  http://www.ncbi.nlm.nih.gov/entrez/query.fcgi?cmd=Retrieve&db=pubmed&dopt=Abstract&list_uids=11383926

- **Acne in premature ovarian failure. Reestablishment of cyclic flare-ups with medroxyprogesterone acetate therapy.**
  Author(s): Pochi PE.
  Source: Archives of Dermatology. 1974 April; 109(4): 556-7.
  http://www.ncbi.nlm.nih.gov/entrez/query.fcgi?cmd=Retrieve&db=pubmed&dopt=Abstract&list_uids=4274248

- **Adrenal antibiotics detect asymptomatic auto-immune adrenal insufficiency in young women with premature ovarian failure.**
  Author(s): Merz S.
  Source: Human Reproduction (Oxford, England). 2003 May; 18(5): 1132-3; Author Reply 1133.
  http://www.ncbi.nlm.nih.gov/entrez/query.fcgi?cmd=Retrieve&db=pubmed&dopt=Abstract&list_uids=12721199

- **Adrenal antibodies detect asymptomatic auto-immune adrenal insufficiency in young women with spontaneous premature ovarian failure.**
  Author(s): Bakalov VK, Vanderhoof VH, Bondy CA, Nelson LM.
  Source: Human Reproduction (Oxford, England). 2002 August; 17(8): 2096-100.
  http://www.ncbi.nlm.nih.gov/entrez/query.fcgi?cmd=Retrieve&db=pubmed&dopt=Abstract&list_uids=12151443

- **Aetiology-specific effect of premature ovarian failure on bone mass - is residual ovarian function important?**
  Author(s): Howell SJ, Shalet SM.
  Source: Clinical Endocrinology. 1999 November; 51(5): 531-4.
  http://www.ncbi.nlm.nih.gov/entrez/query.fcgi?cmd=Retrieve&db=pubmed&dopt=Abstract&list_uids=10594512

- **Analysis of peripheral blood lymphocyte subsets, NK cells, and delayed type hypersensitivity skin test in patients with premature ovarian failure.**
  Author(s): Hoek A, van Kasteren Y, de Haan-Meulman M, Hooijkaas H, Schoemaker J, Drexhage HA.
  Source: American Journal of Reproductive Immunology (New York, N.Y. : 1989). 1995 June; 33(6): 495-502.
  http://www.ncbi.nlm.nih.gov/entrez/query.fcgi?cmd=Retrieve&db=pubmed&dopt=Abstract&list_uids=7576124

- **Analysis of the gonadotropin surges in patients with premature ovarian failure undergoing steroid replacement cycles.**
  Author(s): Pellicer A, Matallin P, Valldecabres MC, Miro F, Remohi J.
  Source: Acta Endocrinol (Copenh). 1990 August; 123(2): 149-54.
  http://www.ncbi.nlm.nih.gov/entrez/query.fcgi?cmd=Retrieve&db=pubmed&dopt=Abstract&list_uids=2120876

- **Androgen serum levels in women with premature ovarian failure compared to fertile and menopausal controls.**
  Author(s): Hartmann BW, Kirchengast S, Albrecht A, Laml T, Soregi G, Huber JC.
  Source: Gynecologic and Obstetric Investigation. 1997; 44(2): 127-31.
  http://www.ncbi.nlm.nih.gov/entrez/query.fcgi?cmd=Retrieve&db=pubmed&dopt=Abstract&list_uids=9286728

- **Anti-nuclear antibodies in patients with premature ovarian failure.**
  Author(s): Ishizuka B, Kudo Y, Amemiya A, Yamada H, Matsuda T, Ogata T.
  Source: Human Reproduction (Oxford, England). 1999 January; 14(1): 70-5.
  http://www.ncbi.nlm.nih.gov/entrez/query.fcgi?cmd=Retrieve&db=pubmed&dopt=Abstract&list_uids=10374097

- **Antiovarian antibody in premature ovarian failure.**
  Author(s): Chattopadhyay D, Sen MR, Katiyar P, Pandey LK.
  Source: Indian Journal of Medical Sciences. 1999 June; 53(6): 254-8.
  http://www.ncbi.nlm.nih.gov/entrez/query.fcgi?cmd=Retrieve&db=pubmed&dopt=Abstract&list_uids=10776506

- **Aromatic hydrocarbon receptor-driven Bax gene expression is required for premature ovarian failure caused by biohazardous environmental chemicals.**
  Author(s): Matikainen T, Perez GI, Jurisicova A, Pru JK, Schlezinger JJ, Ryu HY, Laine J, Sakai T, Korsmeyer SJ, Casper RF, Sherr DH, Tilly JL.
  Source: Nature Genetics. 2001 August; 28(4): 355-60.
  http://www.ncbi.nlm.nih.gov/entrez/query.fcgi?cmd=Retrieve&db=pubmed&dopt=Abstract&list_uids=11455387

- **Association between idiopathic premature ovarian failure and fragile X premutation.**
  Author(s): Marozzi A, Vegetti W, Manfredini E, Tibiletti MG, Testa G, Crosignani PG, Ginelli E, Meneveri R, Dalpra L.
  Source: Human Reproduction (Oxford, England). 2000 January; 15(1): 197-202.
  http://www.ncbi.nlm.nih.gov/entrez/query.fcgi?cmd=Retrieve&db=pubmed&dopt=Abstract&list_uids=10611212

- **Association of premature ovarian failure with HLA antigens.**
  Author(s): Walfish PG, Gottesman IS, Shewchuk AB, Bain J, Hawe BS, Farid NR.
  Source: Tissue Antigens. 1983 February; 21(2): 168-9.
  http://www.ncbi.nlm.nih.gov/entrez/query.fcgi?cmd=Retrieve&db=pubmed&dopt=Abstract&list_uids=6601866

- **Autoantibodies to steroidogenic enzymes in autoimmune polyglandular syndrome, Addison's disease, and premature ovarian failure.**
  Author(s): Chen S, Sawicka J, Betterle C, Powell M, Prentice L, Volpato M, Rees Smith B, Furmaniak J.
  Source: The Journal of Clinical Endocrinology and Metabolism. 1996 May; 81(5): 1871-6.
  http://www.ncbi.nlm.nih.gov/entrez/query.fcgi?cmd=Retrieve&db=pubmed&dopt=Abstract&list_uids=8626850

- **Autoantibodies to steroidogenic enzymes in patients with premature ovarian failure with and without Addison's disease.**
  Author(s): Dal Pra C, Chen S, Furmaniak J, Smith BR, Pedini B, Moscon A, Zanchetta R, Betterle C.
  Source: European Journal of Endocrinology / European Federation of Endocrine Societies. 2003 May; 148(5): 565-70.
  http://www.ncbi.nlm.nih.gov/entrez/query.fcgi?cmd=Retrieve&db=pubmed&dopt=Abstract&list_uids=12720541

- **Autoimmune etiology in premature ovarian failure.**
  Author(s): LaBarbera AR, Miller MM, Ober C, Rebar RW.
  Source: Am J Reprod Immunol Microbiol. 1988 March; 16(3): 115-22. Review. No Abstract Available.
  http://www.ncbi.nlm.nih.gov/entrez/query.fcgi?cmd=Retrieve&db=pubmed&dopt=Abstract&list_uids=3289410

- **Autoimmune premature ovarian failure with polyendocrinopathy and spontaneous recovery of ovarian follicular activity.**
  Author(s): Tan SL, Hague WM, Becker F, Jacobs HS.
  Source: Fertility and Sterility. 1986 March; 45(3): 421-4.
  http://www.ncbi.nlm.nih.gov/entrez/query.fcgi?cmd=Retrieve&db=pubmed&dopt=Abstract&list_uids=3949043

- **Autoimmune premature ovarian failure.**
  Author(s): Kim JG, Moon SY, Chang YS, Lee JY.
  Source: Journal of Obstetrics and Gynaecology : the Journal of the Institute of Obstetrics and Gynaecology. 1995 February; 21(1): 59-66. Review.
  http://www.ncbi.nlm.nih.gov/entrez/query.fcgi?cmd=Retrieve&db=pubmed&dopt=Abstract&list_uids=8591112

- **Autoimmune premature ovarian failure: of mice and women.**
  Author(s): Kalantaridou SN, Nelson LM.
  Source: J Am Med Womens Assoc. 1998 Winter; 53(1): 18-20. Review.
  http://www.ncbi.nlm.nih.gov/entrez/query.fcgi?cmd=Retrieve&db=pubmed&dopt=Abstract&list_uids=9458620

- **Autoimmune premature ovarian failure--endocrine aspects of a T cell disease.**
  Author(s): Melner MH, Feltus FA.
  Source: Endocrinology. 1999 August; 140(8): 3401-3. Review.
  http://www.ncbi.nlm.nih.gov/entrez/query.fcgi?cmd=Retrieve&db=pubmed&dopt=Abstract&list_uids=10433192

- **Autoimmunity in premature ovarian failure.**
  Author(s): Muechler EK, Huang KE, Schenk E.
  Source: Int J Fertil. 1991 March-April; 36(2): 99-103.
  http://www.ncbi.nlm.nih.gov/entrez/query.fcgi?cmd=Retrieve&db=pubmed&dopt=Abstract&list_uids=1674938

- **Autosomal translocation associated with premature ovarian failure.**
  Author(s): Burton KA, Van Ee CC, Purcell K, Winship I, Shelling AN.
  Source: Journal of Medical Genetics. 2000 May; 37(5): E2.
  http://www.ncbi.nlm.nih.gov/entrez/query.fcgi?cmd=Retrieve&db=pubmed&dopt=Abstract&list_uids=10807701

- **Balanced X; 22 translocation in a patient with premature ovarian failure.**
  Author(s): Banerjee N, Kriplani A, Takkar D, Kucheria K.
  Source: Acta Genet Med Gemellol (Roma). 1997; 46(4): 241-4.
  http://www.ncbi.nlm.nih.gov/entrez/query.fcgi?cmd=Retrieve&db=pubmed&dopt=Abstract&list_uids=9862012

- **Biological bases of premature ovarian failure.**
  Author(s): Gosden RG, Faddy MJ.
  Source: Reproduction, Fertility, and Development. 1998; 10(1): 73-8. Review.
  http://www.ncbi.nlm.nih.gov/entrez/query.fcgi?cmd=Retrieve&db=pubmed&dopt=Abstract&list_uids=9727595

- **Bone loss in young women with karyotypically normal spontaneous premature ovarian failure.**
  Author(s): Anasti JN, Kalantaridou SN, Kimzey LM, Defensor RA, Nelson LM.
  Source: Obstetrics and Gynecology. 1998 January; 91(1): 12-5.
  http://www.ncbi.nlm.nih.gov/entrez/query.fcgi?cmd=Retrieve&db=pubmed&dopt=Abstract&list_uids=9464713

- **Case report. Successive pregnancies in a patient with premature ovarian failure.**
  Author(s): Nakai M, Tatsumi H, Arai M.
  Source: European Journal of Obstetrics, Gynecology, and Reproductive Biology. 1984 November; 18(4): 217-24.
  http://www.ncbi.nlm.nih.gov/entrez/query.fcgi?cmd=Retrieve&db=pubmed&dopt=Abstract&list_uids=6440817

- **Case report: spontaneous pregnancy following thymectomy for myasthenia gravis associated with premature ovarian failure.**
  Author(s): Chung TK, Haines CJ, Yip SK.
  Source: Asia Oceania J Obstet Gynaecol. 1993 September; 19(3): 253-5.
  http://www.ncbi.nlm.nih.gov/entrez/query.fcgi?cmd=Retrieve&db=pubmed&dopt=Abstract&list_uids=8250758

- **Case-control study on risk factors for premature ovarian failure.**
  Author(s): Testa G, Chiaffarino F, Vegetti W, Nicolosi A, Caliari I, Alagna F, Bolis PF, Parazzini F, Crosignani PG.
  Source: Gynecologic and Obstetric Investigation. 2001; 51(1): 40-3.
  http://www.ncbi.nlm.nih.gov/entrez/query.fcgi?cmd=Retrieve&db=pubmed&dopt=Abstract&list_uids=11150874

- **Characterization of idiopathic premature ovarian failure.**
  Author(s): Conway GS, Kaltsas G, Patel A, Davies MC, Jacobs HS.
  Source: Fertility and Sterility. 1996 February; 65(2): 337-41.
  http://www.ncbi.nlm.nih.gov/entrez/query.fcgi?cmd=Retrieve&db=pubmed&dopt=Abstract&list_uids=8566258

- **Chemotherapy-induced premature ovarian failure: mechanisms and prevention.**
  Author(s): Ataya K, Moghissi K.
  Source: Steroids. 1989 December; 54(6): 607-26.
  http://www.ncbi.nlm.nih.gov/entrez/query.fcgi?cmd=Retrieve&db=pubmed&dopt=Abstract&list_uids=2558431

- **Circulating antiovarian antibodies in premature ovarian failure.**
  Author(s): Alper MM, Garner PR.
  Source: Obstetrics and Gynecology. 1987 July; 70(1): 144.
  http://www.ncbi.nlm.nih.gov/entrez/query.fcgi?cmd=Retrieve&db=pubmed&dopt=Abstract&list_uids=3601264

- **Circulating antiovarian antibodies in premature ovarian failure.**
  Author(s): Damewood MD, Zacur HA, Hoffman GJ, Rock JA.
  Source: Obstetrics and Gynecology. 1986 December; 68(6): 850-4.
  http://www.ncbi.nlm.nih.gov/entrez/query.fcgi?cmd=Retrieve&db=pubmed&dopt=Abstract&list_uids=3537879

- **Circulating tumor necrosis factor (TNF)-alpha in normally cycling women and patients with premature ovarian failure and polycystic ovaries.**
  Author(s): Naz RK, Thurston D, Santoro N.
  Source: American Journal of Reproductive Immunology (New York, N.Y. : 1989). 1995 September; 34(3): 170-5.
  http://www.ncbi.nlm.nih.gov/entrez/query.fcgi?cmd=Retrieve&db=pubmed&dopt=Abstract&list_uids=8561874

- **Comparison of transdermal to oral estradiol administration on hormonal and hepatic parameters in women with premature ovarian failure.**
  Author(s): Steingold KA, Matt DW, DeZiegler D, Sealey JE, Fratkin M, Reznikov S.
  Source: The Journal of Clinical Endocrinology and Metabolism. 1991 August; 73(2): 275-80.
  http://www.ncbi.nlm.nih.gov/entrez/query.fcgi?cmd=Retrieve&db=pubmed&dopt=Abstract&list_uids=1906893

- **Corticosteroids do not influence ovarian responsiveness to gonadotropins in patients with premature ovarian failure: a randomized, placebo-controlled trial.**
  Author(s): van Kasteren YM, Braat DD, Hemrika DJ, Lambalk CB, Rekers-Momrabg LT, von Blomberg BM, Schoemaker J.
  Source: Fertility and Sterility. 1999 January; 71(1): 90-5.
  http://www.ncbi.nlm.nih.gov/entrez/query.fcgi?cmd=Retrieve&db=pubmed&dopt=Abstract&list_uids=9935122

- **Cyclic steroid replacement alters auditory brainstem responses in young women with premature ovarian failure.**
  Author(s): Elkind-Hirsch KE, Wallace E, Stach BA, Jerger JF.
  Source: Hearing Research. 1992 December; 64(1): 93-8.
  http://www.ncbi.nlm.nih.gov/entrez/query.fcgi?cmd=Retrieve&db=pubmed&dopt=Abstract&list_uids=1490905

- **Cyclic therapy resulted in pregnancy in premature ovarian failure.**
  Author(s): Ohsawa M, Wu MC, Masahashi T, Asai M, Narita O.
  Source: Obstetrics and Gynecology. 1985 September; 66(3 Suppl): 64S-67S.
  http://www.ncbi.nlm.nih.gov/entrez/query.fcgi?cmd=Retrieve&db=pubmed&dopt=Abstract&list_uids=2410842

- **Cytogenetic studies in premature ovarian failure.**
  Author(s): Boczkowski K, Radwanska E, Weintraub L, Herman E, Teter J.
  Source: American Journal of Obstetrics and Gynecology. 1969 June 15; 104(4): 594-5.
  http://www.ncbi.nlm.nih.gov/entrez/query.fcgi?cmd=Retrieve&db=pubmed&dopt=Abstract&list_uids=5786708

- **De novo deletion of Xq associated with premature ovarian failure.**
  Author(s): McAuley K, Cambridge L, Galloway S, Sullivan J, Manning P.
  Source: Aust N Z J Med. 2000 February; 30(1): 89-90. No Abstract Available.
  http://www.ncbi.nlm.nih.gov/entrez/query.fcgi?cmd=Retrieve&db=pubmed&dopt=Abstract&list_uids=10800888

- **Detection of anti-ovarian antibodies by indirect immunofluorescence in patients with premature ovarian failure.**
  Author(s): Kirsop R, Brock CR, Robinson BG, Baber RJ, Wells JV, Saunders DM.
  Source: Reproduction, Fertility, and Development. 1991; 3(5): 537-41.
  http://www.ncbi.nlm.nih.gov/entrez/query.fcgi?cmd=Retrieve&db=pubmed&dopt=Abstract&list_uids=1788393

- **Determination of the steroidogenic capacity in premature ovarian failure.**
  Author(s): Bermudez JA, Moran C, Herrera J, Barahona E, Perez MC, Zarate A.
  Source: Fertility and Sterility. 1993 October; 60(4): 668-71.
  http://www.ncbi.nlm.nih.gov/entrez/query.fcgi?cmd=Retrieve&db=pubmed&dopt=Abstract&list_uids=8405522

- **Development of a radioligand receptor assay for measuring follitropin in serum: application to premature ovarian failure.**
  Author(s): Schneyer AL, Sluss PM, Whitcomb RW, Hall JE, Crowley WF Jr, Freeman RG.
  Source: Clinical Chemistry. 1991 April; 37(4): 508-14.
  http://www.ncbi.nlm.nih.gov/entrez/query.fcgi?cmd=Retrieve&db=pubmed&dopt=Abstract&list_uids=1901773

- **Development of luteinized graafian follicles in patients with karyotypically normal spontaneous premature ovarian failure.**
  Author(s): Nelson LM, Anasti JN, Kimzey LM, Defensor RA, Lipetz KJ, White BJ, Shawker TH, Merino MJ.
  Source: The Journal of Clinical Endocrinology and Metabolism. 1994 November; 79(5): 1470-5.
  http://www.ncbi.nlm.nih.gov/entrez/query.fcgi?cmd=Retrieve&db=pubmed&dopt=Abstract&list_uids=7962345

- **Dicentric isochromosome X with premature ovarian failure: report of two cases.**
  Author(s): Wu MH, Tzeng CC, Kuo PL.
  Source: J Formos Med Assoc. 1993 September; 92(9): 848-50.
  http://www.ncbi.nlm.nih.gov/entrez/query.fcgi?cmd=Retrieve&db=pubmed&dopt=Abstract&list_uids=7904872

- **Does gonadotropin suppression result in follicular development in premature ovarian failure?**
  Author(s): Buckler HM, Healy DL, Burger HG.
  Source: Gynecological Endocrinology : the Official Journal of the International Society of Gynecological Endocrinology. 1993 June; 7(2): 123-8.
  http://www.ncbi.nlm.nih.gov/entrez/query.fcgi?cmd=Retrieve&db=pubmed&dopt=Abstract&list_uids=8213226

- **Donation of oocytes as treatment for infertility in patients with premature ovarian failure. Awarded the "Nicolau de Moraes Barros" prize for gynecology.**
  Author(s): Franco Junior JG, Baruffi RL, Mauri AL, Pertersen CG, Campos MS, Oliveira JB.
  Source: Sao Paulo Medical Journal = Revista Paulista De Medicina. 1994 January-March; 112(1): 510-6.
  http://www.ncbi.nlm.nih.gov/entrez/query.fcgi?cmd=Retrieve&db=pubmed&dopt=Abstract&list_uids=7871317

- **Dry eye signs and symptoms in women with premature ovarian failure.**
  Author(s): Smith JA, Vitale S, Reed GF, Grieshaber SA, Goodman LA, Vanderhoof VH, Calis KA, Nelson LM.
  Source: Archives of Ophthalmology. 2004 February; 122(2): 151-6.
  http://www.ncbi.nlm.nih.gov/entrez/query.fcgi?cmd=Retrieve&db=pubmed&dopt=Abstract&list_uids=14769589

- **Dynamic hormonal tests in a case of premature ovarian failure.**
  Author(s): Asch RH, Bryner J, Watatani H, Mills T, Greenblatt RB.
  Source: Southern Medical Journal. 1979 January; 72(1): 72-4.
  http://www.ncbi.nlm.nih.gov/entrez/query.fcgi?cmd=Retrieve&db=pubmed&dopt=Abstract&list_uids=760227

- **Dysfunction of monocytes and dendritic cells in patients with premature ovarian failure.**
  Author(s): Hoek A, van Kasteren Y, de Haan-Meulman M, Schoemaker J, Drexhage HA.
  Source: American Journal of Reproductive Immunology (New York, N.Y. : 1989). 1993 December; 30(4): 207-17.
  http://www.ncbi.nlm.nih.gov/entrez/query.fcgi?cmd=Retrieve&db=pubmed&dopt=Abstract&list_uids=8129847

- **Effect of hormone replacement therapy on growth hormone stimulation in women with premature ovarian failure.**
  Author(s): Hartmann BW, Kirchengast S, Albrecht A, Huber JC, Soregi G.
  Source: Fertility and Sterility. 1997 July; 68(1): 103-7.Erratum In: Fertil Steril 1997 October; 68(4): 749-50.
  http://www.ncbi.nlm.nih.gov/entrez/query.fcgi?cmd=Retrieve&db=pubmed&dopt=Abstract&list_uids=9207592

- **Effect of hormone replacement therapy on spinal bone mineral density and T lymphocyte subsets in premature ovarian failure and Turner's syndrome.**
  Author(s): Kurabayashi T, Yasuda M, Fujimaki T, Yamamoto Y, Oda K, Tanaka K.
  Source: International Journal of Gynaecology and Obstetrics: the Official Organ of the International Federation of Gynaecology and Obstetrics. 1993 July; 42(1): 25-31.
  http://www.ncbi.nlm.nih.gov/entrez/query.fcgi?cmd=Retrieve&db=pubmed&dopt=Abstract&list_uids=8103471

- **Effect on plasma gonadotropins of cyclic steroid replacement in women with premature ovarian failure.**
  Author(s): Lutjen PJ, Findlay JK, Trounson AO, Leeton JF, Chan LK.
  Source: The Journal of Clinical Endocrinology and Metabolism. 1986 February; 62(2): 419-23.
  http://www.ncbi.nlm.nih.gov/entrez/query.fcgi?cmd=Retrieve&db=pubmed&dopt=Abstract&list_uids=3079776

- **Eleven X chromosome breakpoints associated with premature ovarian failure (POF) map to a 15-Mb YAC contig spanning Xq21.**
  Author(s): Sala C, Arrigo G, Torri G, Martinazzi F, Riva P, Larizza L, Philippe C, Jonveaux P, Sloan F, Labella T, Toniolo D.
  Source: Genomics. 1997 February 15; 40(1): 123-31.
  http://www.ncbi.nlm.nih.gov/entrez/query.fcgi?cmd=Retrieve&db=pubmed&dopt=Abstract&list_uids=9070928

- **Endocrinological findings in two patients with premature ovarian failure.**
  Author(s): Adamopoulos DA, Loraine JA.
  Source: Lancet. 1971 January 23; 1(7691): 161-3.
  http://www.ncbi.nlm.nih.gov/entrez/query.fcgi?cmd=Retrieve&db=pubmed&dopt=Abstract&list_uids=4102186

- **Endometrial blood flow response to hormone replacement therapy in women with premature ovarian failure: a transvaginal Doppler study.**
  Author(s): Achiron R, Levran D, Sivan E, Lipitz S, Dor J, Mashiach S.
  Source: Fertility and Sterility. 1995 March; 63(3): 550-4.
  http://www.ncbi.nlm.nih.gov/entrez/query.fcgi?cmd=Retrieve&db=pubmed&dopt=Abstract&list_uids=7851585

- **Evidence for a genetic factor in the etiology of premature ovarian failure.**
  Author(s): Coulam CB, Stringfellow S, Hoefnagel D.
  Source: Fertility and Sterility. 1983 November; 40(5): 693-5.
  http://www.ncbi.nlm.nih.gov/entrez/query.fcgi?cmd=Retrieve&db=pubmed&dopt=Abstract&list_uids=6628716

- **Experience with a 'physiological' steroid replacement regimen for the establishment of a receptive endometrium in women with premature ovarian failure.**
  Author(s): Critchley HO, Buckley CH, Anderson DC.
  Source: British Journal of Obstetrics and Gynaecology. 1990 September; 97(9): 804-10.
  http://www.ncbi.nlm.nih.gov/entrez/query.fcgi?cmd=Retrieve&db=pubmed&dopt=Abstract&list_uids=2242365

- **Extraovarian endocrine abnormalities in north Indian women with premature ovarian failure.**
  Author(s): Shah A, Mithal A, Bhatia E, Godbole MM.
  Source: Natl Med J India. 1995 January-February; 8(1): 9-12.
  http://www.ncbi.nlm.nih.gov/entrez/query.fcgi?cmd=Retrieve&db=pubmed&dopt=Abstract&list_uids=7696955

- **Failure to identify heterozygotes for galactosaemia in women with premature ovarian failure.**
  Author(s): Fraser IS, Shearman RP, Wilcken B, Brown A, Davis K.
  Source: Lancet. 1987 September 5; 2(8558): 566.
  http://www.ncbi.nlm.nih.gov/entrez/query.fcgi?cmd=Retrieve&db=pubmed&dopt=Abstract&list_uids=2887854

- **Familial idiopathic premature ovarian failure: an overrated and underestimated genetic disease?**
  Author(s): van Kasteren YM, Hundscheid RD, Smits AP, Cremers FP, van Zonneveld P, Braat DD.
  Source: Human Reproduction (Oxford, England). 1999 October; 14(10): 2455-9.
  http://www.ncbi.nlm.nih.gov/entrez/query.fcgi?cmd=Retrieve&db=pubmed&dopt=Abstract&list_uids=10527968

- **Familial premature ovarian failure due to an interstitial deletion of the long arm of the X chromosome.**
  Author(s): Krauss CM, Turksoy RN, Atkins L, McLaughlin C, Brown LG, Page DC.
  Source: The New England Journal of Medicine. 1987 July 16; 317(3): 125-31.
  http://www.ncbi.nlm.nih.gov/entrez/query.fcgi?cmd=Retrieve&db=pubmed&dopt=Abstract&list_uids=3600701

- **Familial premature ovarian failure.**
  Author(s): Mattison DR, Evans MI, Schwimmer WB, White BJ, Jensen B, Schulman JD.
  Source: American Journal of Human Genetics. 1984 November; 36(6): 1341-8.
  http://www.ncbi.nlm.nih.gov/entrez/query.fcgi?cmd=Retrieve&db=pubmed&dopt=Abstract&list_uids=6517055

- **Female carriers of fragile X premutations have no increased risk for additional diseases other than premature ovarian failure.**
  Author(s): Hundscheid RD, Smits AP, Thomas CM, Kiemeney LA, Braat DD.
  Source: American Journal of Medical Genetics. 2003 February 15; 117A(1): 6-9.
  http://www.ncbi.nlm.nih.gov/entrez/query.fcgi?cmd=Retrieve&db=pubmed&dopt=Abstract&list_uids=12548733

- **Female sex preponderance for idiopathic familial premature ovarian failure suggests an X chromosome defect: opinion.**
  Author(s): Davis CJ, Davison RM, Payne NN, Rodeck CH, Conway GS.
  Source: Human Reproduction (Oxford, England). 2000 November; 15(11): 2418-22. Review.
  http://www.ncbi.nlm.nih.gov/entrez/query.fcgi?cmd=Retrieve&db=pubmed&dopt=Abstract&list_uids=11056145

- **First reported convergence of premature ovarian failure and cutis marmorata telangiectatica congenita.**
  Author(s): Sills ES, Harmon KE, Tucker MJ.
  Source: Fertility and Sterility. 2002 December; 78(6): 1314-6. Review
  http://www.ncbi.nlm.nih.gov/entrez/query.fcgi?cmd=Retrieve&db=pubmed&dopt=Abstract&list_uids=12477531

- **FISH characterization of the Xq21 breakpoint in a translocation carrier with premature ovarian failure.**
  Author(s): Riva P, Magnani I, Fuhrmann Conti AM, Gelli D, Sala C, Toniolo D, Larizza L.
  Source: Clinical Genetics. 1996 October; 50(4): 267-9.
  http://www.ncbi.nlm.nih.gov/entrez/query.fcgi?cmd=Retrieve&db=pubmed&dopt=Abstract&list_uids=9001815

- **Follicle-stimulating hormone beta gene structure in premature ovarian failure.**
  Author(s): Layman LC, Shelley ME, Huey LO, Wall SW, Tho SP, McDonough PG.
  Source: Fertility and Sterility. 1993 November; 60(5): 852-7.
  http://www.ncbi.nlm.nih.gov/entrez/query.fcgi?cmd=Retrieve&db=pubmed&dopt=Abstract&list_uids=8224270

- **Follicle-stimulating hormone receptor gene mutations are rare in Japanese women with premature ovarian failure and polycystic ovary syndrome.**
  Author(s): Takakura K, Takebayashi K, Wang HQ, Kimura F, Kasahara K, Noda Y.
  Source: Fertility and Sterility. 2001 January; 75(1): 207-9.
  http://www.ncbi.nlm.nih.gov/entrez/query.fcgi?cmd=Retrieve&db=pubmed&dopt=Abstract&list_uids=11163840

- **Fragile X premutation in women with sporadic premature ovarian failure in Slovenia.**
  Author(s): Gersak K, Meden-Vrtovec H, Peterlin B.
  Source: Human Reproduction (Oxford, England). 2003 August; 18(8): 1637-40.
  http://www.ncbi.nlm.nih.gov/entrez/query.fcgi?cmd=Retrieve&db=pubmed&dopt=Abstract&list_uids=12871874

- **Fragile X premutation is a significant risk factor for premature ovarian failure: the International Collaborative POF in Fragile X study--preliminary data.**
  Author(s): Allingham-Hawkins DJ, Babul-Hirji R, Chitayat D, Holden JJ, Yang KT, Lee C, Hudson R, Gorwill H, Nolin SL, Glicksman A, Jenkins EC, Brown WT, Howard-Peebles PN, Becchi C, Cummings E, Fallon L, Seitz S, Black SH, Vianna-Morgante AM, Costa SS, Otto PA, Mingroni-Netto RC, Murray A, Webb J, Vieri F.
  Source: American Journal of Medical Genetics. 1999 April 2; 83(4): 322-5.
  http://www.ncbi.nlm.nih.gov/entrez/query.fcgi?cmd=Retrieve&db=pubmed&dopt=Abstract&list_uids=10208170

- **Fragile X premutation screening in women with premature ovarian failure.**
  Author(s): Conway GS, Payne NN, Webb J, Murray A, Jacobs PA.
  Source: Human Reproduction (Oxford, England). 1998 May; 13(5): 1184-7.
  http://www.ncbi.nlm.nih.gov/entrez/query.fcgi?cmd=Retrieve&db=pubmed&dopt=Abstract&list_uids=9647544

- **Fragile X premutations in familial premature ovarian failure.**
  Author(s): Conway GS, Hettiarachchi S, Murray A, Jacobs PA.
  Source: Lancet. 1995 July 29; 346(8970): 309-10.
  http://www.ncbi.nlm.nih.gov/entrez/query.fcgi?cmd=Retrieve&db=pubmed&dopt=Abstract&list_uids=7630263

- **FRAXA premutation associated with premature ovarian failure.**
  Author(s): Vianna-Morgante AM, Costa SS, Pares AS, Verreschi IT.
  Source: American Journal of Medical Genetics. 1996 August 9; 64(2): 373-5.
  http://www.ncbi.nlm.nih.gov/entrez/query.fcgi?cmd=Retrieve&db=pubmed&dopt=Abstract&list_uids=8844084

- **FRAXA premutations are not a cause of familial premature ovarian failure.**
  Author(s): Marozzi A, Dalpra L, Ginelli E, Tibiletti MG, Crosignani PG.
  Source: Human Reproduction (Oxford, England). 1999 February; 14(2): 573-5.
  http://www.ncbi.nlm.nih.gov/entrez/query.fcgi?cmd=Retrieve&db=pubmed&dopt=Abstract&list_uids=10100016

- **G769A variation of inhibin alpha-gene in korean women with premature ovarian failure.**
  Author(s): Jeong HJ, Cho SW, Kim HA, Lee SH, Cho JH, Choi DH, Kwon H, Cha WT, Han JE, Cha KY.
  Source: Yonsei Medical Journal. 2004 June 30; 45(3): 479-82.
  http://www.ncbi.nlm.nih.gov/entrez/query.fcgi?cmd=Retrieve&db=pubmed&dopt=Abstract&list_uids=15227735

- **Gamete intra fallopian transfer (GIFT) and oocyte donation--a novel treatment for infertility in premature ovarian failure.**
  Author(s): Asch RH, Balmaceda JP, Ord T, Borrero C, Rodriguez Rigau LJ, Rojas FJ.
  Source: Gynecological Endocrinology : the Official Journal of the International Society of Gynecological Endocrinology. 1987 March; 1(1): 105-11.
  http://www.ncbi.nlm.nih.gov/entrez/query.fcgi?cmd=Retrieve&db=pubmed&dopt=Abstract&list_uids=2459900

- **Gamete intrafallopian transfer in premature ovarian failure.**
  Author(s): Li TC.
  Source: Fertility and Sterility. 1988 November; 50(5): 831-2.
  http://www.ncbi.nlm.nih.gov/entrez/query.fcgi?cmd=Retrieve&db=pubmed&dopt=Abstract&list_uids=3181499

- **Genes and premature ovarian failure.**
  Author(s): Christin-Maitre S, Vasseur C, Portnoi MF, Bouchard P.
  Source: Molecular and Cellular Endocrinology. 1998 October 25; 145(1-2): 75-80. Review.
  http://www.ncbi.nlm.nih.gov/entrez/query.fcgi?cmd=Retrieve&db=pubmed&dopt=Abstract&list_uids=9922102

- **Genetic disorders in premature ovarian failure.**
  Author(s): Laml T, Preyer O, Umek W, Hengstschlager M, Hanzal H.
  Source: Human Reproduction Update. 2002 September-October; 8(5): 483-91. Review.
  http://www.ncbi.nlm.nih.gov/entrez/query.fcgi?cmd=Retrieve&db=pubmed&dopt=Abstract&list_uids=12398227

- **Genomic organization and polymorphism of human angiotensin II type 2 receptor: no evidence for its gene mutation in two families of human premature ovarian failure syndrome.**
  Author(s): Katsuya T, Horiuchi M, Minami S, Koike G, Santoro NF, Hsueh AJ, Dzau VJ.
  Source: Molecular and Cellular Endocrinology. 1997 March 28; 127(2): 221-8.
  http://www.ncbi.nlm.nih.gov/entrez/query.fcgi?cmd=Retrieve&db=pubmed&dopt=Abstract&list_uids=9099917

- **Gonadotropin suppression for the treatment of karyotypically normal spontaneous premature ovarian failure: a controlled trial.**
  Author(s): Nelson LM, Kimzey LM, White BJ, Merriam GR.
  Source: Fertility and Sterility. 1992 January; 57(1): 50-5.
  http://www.ncbi.nlm.nih.gov/entrez/query.fcgi?cmd=Retrieve&db=pubmed&dopt=Abstract&list_uids=1730330

- **Gonadotropin-induced pregnancy following "premature ovarian failure".**
  Author(s): Johnson TR Jr, Peterson EP.
  Source: Fertility and Sterility. 1979 March; 31(3): 351-2.
  http://www.ncbi.nlm.nih.gov/entrez/query.fcgi?cmd=Retrieve&db=pubmed&dopt=Abstract&list_uids=437172

- **Gynaecography in premature ovarian failure and ovarian dysgenesis.**
  Author(s): Kreel L, Ginsburg J, Green MF.
  Source: British Medical Journal. 1969 March 15; 1(645): 682-6.
  http://www.ncbi.nlm.nih.gov/entrez/query.fcgi?cmd=Retrieve&db=pubmed&dopt=Abstract&list_uids=5774319

- **High levels of serum allopregnanolone in women with premature ovarian failure.**
  Author(s): Bernardi F, Hartmann B, Casarosa E, Luisi S, Stomati M, Fadalti M, Florio P, Santuz M, Luisi M, Petraglia F, Genazzani AR.
  Source: Gynecological Endocrinology : the Official Journal of the International Society of Gynecological Endocrinology. 1998 October; 12(5): 339-45.
  http://www.ncbi.nlm.nih.gov/entrez/query.fcgi?cmd=Retrieve&db=pubmed&dopt=Abstract&list_uids=9859027

- **High-dose, short-term glucocorticoids for the treatment of infertility resulting from premature ovarian failure.**
  Author(s): Corenblum B, Rowe T, Taylor PJ.
  Source: Fertility and Sterility. 1993 May; 59(5): 988-91.
  http://www.ncbi.nlm.nih.gov/entrez/query.fcgi?cmd=Retrieve&db=pubmed&dopt=Abstract&list_uids=8486200

- **Homologous telomere association of 19q in a female with premature ovarian failure.**
  Author(s): Zahed L, Darwiche N, Batanian JR, Awwad J.
  Source: Clinical Genetics. 2002 October; 62(4): 310-4.
  http://www.ncbi.nlm.nih.gov/entrez/query.fcgi?cmd=Retrieve&db=pubmed&dopt=Abstract&list_uids=12372059

- **Hormone replacement therapy alters insulin sensitivity in young women with premature ovarian failure.**
  Author(s): Elkind-Hirsch KE, Sherman LD, Malinak R.
  Source: The Journal of Clinical Endocrinology and Metabolism. 1993 February; 76(2): 472-5.
  http://www.ncbi.nlm.nih.gov/entrez/query.fcgi?cmd=Retrieve&db=pubmed&dopt=Abstract&list_uids=8432792

- **Human leukocyte antigen typing and associated abnormalities in premature ovarian failure.**
  Author(s): Jaroudi KA, Arora M, Sheth KV, Sieck UV, Willemsen WN.
  Source: Human Reproduction (Oxford, England). 1994 November; 9(11): 2006-9.
  http://www.ncbi.nlm.nih.gov/entrez/query.fcgi?cmd=Retrieve&db=pubmed&dopt=Abstract&list_uids=7868665

- **Human leukocyte antigen-DQB1* genotypes encoding aspartate at position 57 are associated with 3beta-hydroxysteroid dehydrogenase autoimmunity in premature ovarian failure.**
  Author(s): Arif S, Underhill JA, Donaldson P, Conway GS, Peakman M.
  Source: The Journal of Clinical Endocrinology and Metabolism. 1999 March; 84(3): 1056-60.
  http://www.ncbi.nlm.nih.gov/entrez/query.fcgi?cmd=Retrieve&db=pubmed&dopt=Abstract&list_uids=10084595

- **Hypergonadotropic amenorrhea and premature ovarian failure: a review.**
  Author(s): Rebar RW.
  Source: J Reprod Med. 1982 April; 27(4): 179-86. Review.
  http://www.ncbi.nlm.nih.gov/entrez/query.fcgi?cmd=Retrieve&db=pubmed&dopt=Abstract&list_uids=6808131

- **Identification of novel mutations in FOXL2 associated with premature ovarian failure.**
  Author(s): Harris SE, Chand AL, Winship IM, Gersak K, Aittomaki K, Shelling AN.
  Source: Molecular Human Reproduction. 2002 August; 8(8): 729-33.
  http://www.ncbi.nlm.nih.gov/entrez/query.fcgi?cmd=Retrieve&db=pubmed&dopt=Abstract&list_uids=12149404

- **Identification of ovarian antibodies by immunofluorescence, enzyme-linked immunosorbent assay or immunoblotting in premature ovarian failure.**
  Author(s): Wheatcroft NJ, Salt C, Milford-Ward A, Cooke ID, Weetman AP.
  Source: Human Reproduction (Oxford, England). 1997 December; 12(12): 2617-22.
  http://www.ncbi.nlm.nih.gov/entrez/query.fcgi?cmd=Retrieve&db=pubmed&dopt=Abstract&list_uids=9455824

- **Identification of premature ovarian failure patients with underlying autoimmunity.**
  Author(s): Yan G, Schoenfeld D, Penney C, Hurxthal K, Taylor AE, Faustman D.
  Source: Journal of Women's Health & Gender-Based Medicine. 2000 April; 9(3): 275-87.
  http://www.ncbi.nlm.nih.gov/entrez/query.fcgi?cmd=Retrieve&db=pubmed&dopt=Abstract&list_uids=10787223

- **Idiopathic premature ovarian failure. A clinical and biochemical study.**
  Author(s): Naidoo C, Norman RJ, Khatree M, Joubert SM.
  Source: South African Medical Journal. Suid-Afrikaanse Tydskrif Vir Geneeskunde. 1985 July 20; 68(2): 91-4.
  http://www.ncbi.nlm.nih.gov/entrez/query.fcgi?cmd=Retrieve&db=pubmed&dopt=Abstract&list_uids=3925570

- **Idiopathic premature ovarian failure: clinical and endocrine characteristics.**
  Author(s): Rebar RW, Erickson GF, Yen SS.
  Source: Fertility and Sterility. 1982 January; 37(1): 35-41.
  http://www.ncbi.nlm.nih.gov/entrez/query.fcgi?cmd=Retrieve&db=pubmed&dopt=Abstract&list_uids=6800842

- **Immune disorders in women with premature ovarian failure in initial period.**
  Author(s): Chernyshov VP, Radysh TV, Gura IV, Tatarchuk TP, Khominskaya ZB.
  Source: American Journal of Reproductive Immunology (New York, N.Y. : 1989). 2001 September; 46(3): 220-5.
  http://www.ncbi.nlm.nih.gov/entrez/query.fcgi?cmd=Retrieve&db=pubmed&dopt=Abstract&list_uids=11554695

- **Immunologic studies in patients with premature ovarian failure.**
  Author(s): Ho PC, Tang GW, Fu KH, Fan MC, Lawton JW.
  Source: Obstetrics and Gynecology. 1988 April; 71(4): 622-6.
  http://www.ncbi.nlm.nih.gov/entrez/query.fcgi?cmd=Retrieve&db=pubmed&dopt=Abstract&list_uids=3258418

- **Immunological aspects of premature ovarian failure associated with idiopathic Addison's disease.**
  Author(s): Irvine WJ, Chan MM, Scarth L, Kolb FO, Hartog M, Bayliss RI, Drury MI.
  Source: Lancet. 1968 October 26; 2(7574): 883-7.
  http://www.ncbi.nlm.nih.gov/entrez/query.fcgi?cmd=Retrieve&db=pubmed&dopt=Abstract&list_uids=4176147

- **Immunological disturbances in patients with premature ovarian failure.**
  Author(s): Pekonen F, Siegberg R, Makinen T, Miettinen A, Yli-Korkala O.
  Source: Clinical Endocrinology. 1986 July; 25(1): 1-6.
  http://www.ncbi.nlm.nih.gov/entrez/query.fcgi?cmd=Retrieve&db=pubmed&dopt=Abstract&list_uids=3539415

- **Impaired endothelial function in young women with premature ovarian failure: normalization with hormone therapy.**
  Author(s): Kalantaridou SN, Naka KK, Papanikolaou E, Kazakos N, Kravariti M, Calis KA, Paraskevaidis EA, Sideris DA, Tsatsoulis A, Chrousos GP, Michalis LK.
  Source: The Journal of Clinical Endocrinology and Metabolism. 2004 August; 89(8): 3907-13.
  http://www.ncbi.nlm.nih.gov/entrez/query.fcgi?cmd=Retrieve&db=pubmed&dopt=Abstract&list_uids=15292326

- **Implications of circulating autoantibodies and peripheral blood lymphocyte subsets for the genesis of premature ovarian failure.**
  Author(s): Miyake T, Sato Y, Takeuchi S.
  Source: Journal of Reproductive Immunology. 1987 November; 12(3): 163-71.
  http://www.ncbi.nlm.nih.gov/entrez/query.fcgi?cmd=Retrieve&db=pubmed&dopt=Abstract&list_uids=3123670

- **Imprinting effect in premature ovarian failure confined to paternally inherited fragile X premutations.**
  Author(s): Hundscheid RD, Sistermans EA, Thomas CM, Braat DD, Straatman H, Kiemeney LA, Oostra BA, Smits AP.
  Source: American Journal of Human Genetics. 2000 February; 66(2): 413-8.
  http://www.ncbi.nlm.nih.gov/entrez/query.fcgi?cmd=Retrieve&db=pubmed&dopt=Abstract&list_uids=10677300

- **Incidence of premature ovarian failure.**
  Author(s): Coulam CB, Adamson SC, Annegers JF.
  Source: Obstetrics and Gynecology. 1986 April; 67(4): 604-6.
  http://www.ncbi.nlm.nih.gov/entrez/query.fcgi?cmd=Retrieve&db=pubmed&dopt=Abstract&list_uids=3960433

- **Incipient ovarian failure and premature ovarian failure show the same immunological profile.**
  Author(s): van Kasteren YM, von Blomberg M, Hoek A, de Koning C, Lambalk N, van Montfrans J, Kuik J, Schoemaker J.
  Source: American Journal of Reproductive Immunology (New York, N.Y. : 1989). 2000 June; 43(6): 359-66.
  http://www.ncbi.nlm.nih.gov/entrez/query.fcgi?cmd=Retrieve&db=pubmed&dopt=Abstract&list_uids=10910195

- **Increased peripheral T lymphocyte activation in patients with karyotypically normal spontaneous premature ovarian failure.**
  Author(s): Nelson LM, Kimzey LM, Merriam GR, Fleisher TA.
  Source: Fertility and Sterility. 1991 June; 55(6): 1082-7.
  http://www.ncbi.nlm.nih.gov/entrez/query.fcgi?cmd=Retrieve&db=pubmed&dopt=Abstract&list_uids=2037104

- **Increased prevalence of luteinizing hormone beta-subunit variant in patients with premature ovarian failure.**
  Author(s): Takahashi K, Ozaki T, Okada M, Kurioka H, Kanasaki H, Miyazaki K.
  Source: Fertility and Sterility. 1999 January; 71(1): 96-101.
  http://www.ncbi.nlm.nih.gov/entrez/query.fcgi?cmd=Retrieve&db=pubmed&dopt=Abstract&list_uids=9935123

- **Inheritance in idiopathic premature ovarian failure: analysis of 71 cases.**
  Author(s): Vegetti W, Grazia Tibiletti M, Testa G, de Lauretis Yankowski, Alagna F, Castoldi E, Taborelli M, Motta T, Bolis PF, Dalpra L, Crosignani PG.
  Source: Human Reproduction (Oxford, England). 1998 July; 13(7): 1796-800.
  http://www.ncbi.nlm.nih.gov/entrez/query.fcgi?cmd=Retrieve&db=pubmed&dopt=Abstract&list_uids=9740426

- **Inhibin: a candidate gene for premature ovarian failure.**
  Author(s): Shelling AN, Burton KA, Chand AL, van Ee CC, France JT, Farquhar CM, Milsom SR, Love DR, Gersak K, Aittomaki K, Winship IM.
  Source: Human Reproduction (Oxford, England). 2000 December; 15(12): 2644-9.
  http://www.ncbi.nlm.nih.gov/entrez/query.fcgi?cmd=Retrieve&db=pubmed&dopt=Abstract&list_uids=11098038

- **Is premature ovarian failure an autoimmune disease?**
  Author(s): Wheatcroft N, Weetman AP.
  Source: Autoimmunity. 1997; 25(3): 157-65. Review
  http://www.ncbi.nlm.nih.gov/entrez/query.fcgi?cmd=Retrieve&db=pubmed&dopt=Abstract&list_uids=9272281

- **Karyotypically normal spontaneous premature ovarian failure: evaluation of association with the class II major histocompatibility complex.**
  Author(s): Anasti JN, Adams S, Kimzey LM, Defensor RA, Zachary AA, Nelson LM.
  Source: The Journal of Clinical Endocrinology and Metabolism. 1994 March; 78(3): 722-3.
  http://www.ncbi.nlm.nih.gov/entrez/query.fcgi?cmd=Retrieve&db=pubmed&dopt=Abstract&list_uids=8126148

- **Letter: Premature ovarian failure and the "gonadotropin-resistant" ovary syndrome.**
  Author(s): Goldenberg RL.
  Source: American Journal of Obstetrics and Gynecology. 1975 June 15; 122(4): 539-40.
  http://www.ncbi.nlm.nih.gov/entrez/query.fcgi?cmd=Retrieve&db=pubmed&dopt=Abstract&list_uids=1146916

- **Low molecular weight follicle-stimulating hormone receptor binding inhibitor in sera from premature ovarian failure patients.**
  Author(s): Sluss PM, Schneyer AL.
  Source: The Journal of Clinical Endocrinology and Metabolism. 1992 June; 74(6): 1242-6.
  http://www.ncbi.nlm.nih.gov/entrez/query.fcgi?cmd=Retrieve&db=pubmed&dopt=Abstract&list_uids=1592865

- **Lymphocyte subsets and serum immunoglobulins in patients with premature ovarian failure before and after oestrogen replacement.**
  Author(s): Ho PC, Tang GW, Lawton JW.
  Source: Human Reproduction (Oxford, England). 1993 May; 8(5): 714-6.
  http://www.ncbi.nlm.nih.gov/entrez/query.fcgi?cmd=Retrieve&db=pubmed&dopt=Abstract&list_uids=8314965

- **Mapping of the POF1 locus and identification of putative genes for premature ovarian failure.**
  Author(s): Davison RM, Fox M, Conway GS.
  Source: Molecular Human Reproduction. 2000 April; 6(4): 314-8.
  http://www.ncbi.nlm.nih.gov/entrez/query.fcgi?cmd=Retrieve&db=pubmed&dopt=Abstract&list_uids=10729312

- **Mechanisms of follicular dysfunction in 46,XX spontaneous premature ovarian failure.**
  Author(s): Nelson LM, Bakalov VK.
  Source: Endocrinology and Metabolism Clinics of North America. 2003 September; 32(3): 613-37. Review.
  http://www.ncbi.nlm.nih.gov/entrez/query.fcgi?cmd=Retrieve&db=pubmed&dopt=Abstract&list_uids=14560890

- **Mechanisms of premature ovarian failure.**
  Author(s): Santoro N.
  Source: Annales D'endocrinologie. 2003 April; 64(2): 87-92. Review.
  http://www.ncbi.nlm.nih.gov/entrez/query.fcgi?cmd=Retrieve&db=pubmed&dopt=Abstract&list_uids=12773939

- **Meeting the needs of young women with secondary amenorrhea and spontaneous premature ovarian failure.**
  Author(s): Alzubaidi NH, Chapin HL, Vanderhoof VH, Calis KA, Nelson LM.
  Source: Obstetrics and Gynecology. 2002 May; 99(5 Pt 1): 720-5.
  http://www.ncbi.nlm.nih.gov/entrez/query.fcgi?cmd=Retrieve&db=pubmed&dopt=Abstract&list_uids=11978278

- **Microdeletions in FMR2 may be a significant cause of premature ovarian failure.**
  Author(s): Murray A, Webb J, Dennis N, Conway G, Morton N.
  Source: Journal of Medical Genetics. 1999 October; 36(10): 767-70.
  http://www.ncbi.nlm.nih.gov/entrez/query.fcgi?cmd=Retrieve&db=pubmed&dopt=Abstract&list_uids=10528856

- **Minilaparoscopic ovarian biopsy performed under conscious sedation in women with premature ovarian failure.**
  Author(s): Pellicano M, Zullo F, Cappiello F, Di Carlo C, Cirillo D, Nappi C.
  Source: J Reprod Med. 2000 October; 45(10): 817-22.
  http://www.ncbi.nlm.nih.gov/entrez/query.fcgi?cmd=Retrieve&db=pubmed&dopt=Abstract&list_uids=11077630

- **Molecular analysis of genes on Xp controlling Turner syndrome and premature ovarian failure (POF).**
  Author(s): Zinn AR, Ross JL.
  Source: Seminars in Reproductive Medicine. 2001 June; 19(2): 141-6. Review.
  http://www.ncbi.nlm.nih.gov/entrez/query.fcgi?cmd=Retrieve&db=pubmed&dopt=Abstract&list_uids=11480911

- **Molecular and cytogenetic studies of an X;autosome translocation in a patient with premature ovarian failure and review of the literature.**
  Author(s): Powell CM, Taggart RT, Drumheller TC, Wangsa D, Qian C, Nelson LM, White BJ.
  Source: American Journal of Medical Genetics. 1994 August 1; 52(1): 19-26. Review.
  http://www.ncbi.nlm.nih.gov/entrez/query.fcgi?cmd=Retrieve&db=pubmed&dopt=Abstract&list_uids=7977456

- **Molecular definition of Xq common-deleted region in patients affected by premature ovarian failure.**
  Author(s): Marozzi A, Manfredini E, Tibiletti MG, Furlan D, Villa N, Vegetti W, Crosignani PG, Ginelli E, Meneveri R, Dalpra L.
  Source: Human Genetics. 2000 October; 107(4): 304-11.
  http://www.ncbi.nlm.nih.gov/entrez/query.fcgi?cmd=Retrieve&db=pubmed&dopt=Abstract&list_uids=11129329

- **Most X;autosome translocations associated with premature ovarian failure do not interrupt X-linked genes.**
  Author(s): Prueitt RL, Chen H, Barnes RI, Zinn AR.
  Source: Cytogenetic and Genome Research. 2002; 97(1-2): 32-8.
  http://www.ncbi.nlm.nih.gov/entrez/query.fcgi?cmd=Retrieve&db=pubmed&dopt=Abstract&list_uids=12438735

- **Mutation analysis of the growth differentiation factor-9 and -9B genes in patients with premature ovarian failure and polycystic ovary syndrome.**
  Author(s): Takebayashi K, Takakura K, Wang H, Kimura F, Kasahara K, Noda Y.
  Source: Fertility and Sterility. 2000 November; 74(5): 976-9.
  http://www.ncbi.nlm.nih.gov/entrez/query.fcgi?cmd=Retrieve&db=pubmed&dopt=Abstract&list_uids=11056243

- **Mutation screening and isoform prevalence of the follicle stimulating hormone receptor gene in women with premature ovarian failure, resistant ovary syndrome and polycystic ovary syndrome.**
  Author(s): Conway GS, Conway E, Walker C, Hoppner W, Gromoll J, Simoni M.
  Source: Clinical Endocrinology. 1999 July; 51(1): 97-9.
  http://www.ncbi.nlm.nih.gov/entrez/query.fcgi?cmd=Retrieve&db=pubmed&dopt=Abstract&list_uids=10468971

- **Mutational analysis of the mullerian-inhibiting substance gene and its receptor gene in Japanese women with polycystic ovary syndrome and premature ovarian failure.**
  Author(s): Wang HQ, Takakura K, Takebayashi K, Noda Y.
  Source: Fertility and Sterility. 2002 December; 78(6): 1329-30.
  http://www.ncbi.nlm.nih.gov/entrez/query.fcgi?cmd=Retrieve&db=pubmed&dopt=Abstract&list_uids=12477536

- **Myasthenia gravis and premature ovarian failure.**
  Author(s): Kuki S, Morgan RL, Tucci JR.
  Source: Archives of Internal Medicine. 1981 August; 141(9): 1230-2.
  http://www.ncbi.nlm.nih.gov/entrez/query.fcgi?cmd=Retrieve&db=pubmed&dopt=Abstract&list_uids=6266360

- **Myasthenia gravis and premature ovarian failure.**
  Author(s): Ryan MM, Jones HR Jr.
  Source: Muscle & Nerve. 2004 August; 30(2): 231-3.
  http://www.ncbi.nlm.nih.gov/entrez/query.fcgi?cmd=Retrieve&db=pubmed&dopt=Abstract&list_uids=15266640

- **No evidence for parent of origin influencing premature ovarian failure in fragile X premutation carriers.**
  Author(s): Murray A, Ennis S, Morton N.
  Source: American Journal of Human Genetics. 2000 July; 67(1): 253-4; Author Reply 256-8.
  http://www.ncbi.nlm.nih.gov/entrez/query.fcgi?cmd=Retrieve&db=pubmed&dopt=Abstract&list_uids=10848495

- **No evidence of the inactivating mutation (C566T) in the follicle-stimulating hormone receptor gene in Brazilian women with premature ovarian failure.**
  Author(s): da Fonte Kohek MB, Batista MC, Russell AJ, Vass K, Giacaglia LR, Mendonca BB, Latronico AC.
  Source: Fertility and Sterility. 1998 September; 70(3): 565-7.
  http://www.ncbi.nlm.nih.gov/entrez/query.fcgi?cmd=Retrieve&db=pubmed&dopt=Abstract&list_uids=9757892

- **Oocyte donation and gamete intrafallopian transfer as treatment for premature ovarian failure.**
  Author(s): Asch R, Balmaceda J, Ord T, Borrero C, Cefalu E, Gastaldi C, Rojas F.
  Source: Lancet. 1987 March 21; 1(8534): 687.
  http://www.ncbi.nlm.nih.gov/entrez/query.fcgi?cmd=Retrieve&db=pubmed&dopt=Abstract&list_uids=2882107

- **Oocyte donation and gamete intrafallopian transfer in premature ovarian failure.**
  Author(s): Asch RH, Balmaceda JP, Ord T, Borrero C, Cefalu E, Gastaldi C, Rojas F.
  Source: Fertility and Sterility. 1988 February; 49(2): 263-7.
  http://www.ncbi.nlm.nih.gov/entrez/query.fcgi?cmd=Retrieve&db=pubmed&dopt=Abstract&list_uids=3276563

- **Organ-specific autoimmunity in patients with premature ovarian failure.**
  Author(s): Belvisi L, Bombelli F, Sironi L, Doldi N.
  Source: J Endocrinol Invest. 1993 December; 16(11): 889-92.
  http://www.ncbi.nlm.nih.gov/entrez/query.fcgi?cmd=Retrieve&db=pubmed&dopt=Abstract&list_uids=8144865

- **Ovarian androgen secretion in patients with galactosemia and premature ovarian failure.**
  Author(s): Kaufman FR, Donnell GN, Lobo RA.
  Source: Fertility and Sterility. 1987 June; 47(6): 1033-4.
  http://www.ncbi.nlm.nih.gov/entrez/query.fcgi?cmd=Retrieve&db=pubmed&dopt=Abstract&list_uids=2954857

- **Ovarian antibodies detected by immobilized antigen immunoassay in patients with premature ovarian failure.**
  Author(s): Luborsky JL, Visintin I, Boyers S, Asari T, Caldwell B, DeCherney A.
  Source: The Journal of Clinical Endocrinology and Metabolism. 1990 January; 70(1): 69-75.
  http://www.ncbi.nlm.nih.gov/entrez/query.fcgi?cmd=Retrieve&db=pubmed&dopt=Abstract&list_uids=2104631

- **Ovarian sex cord tumor with annular tubules in a woman with premature ovarian failure.**
  Author(s): Garcia-Galiana S, Monteagudo C, Tortajada M, Llombart A, Cano A.
  Source: Fertility and Sterility. 2001 December; 76(6): 1264-6.
  http://www.ncbi.nlm.nih.gov/entrez/query.fcgi?cmd=Retrieve&db=pubmed&dopt=Abstract&list_uids=11730763

- **Ovarian stimulation in a woman with premature ovarian failure and X-autosome translocation. A case report.**
  Author(s): Causio F, Fischetto R, Leonetti T, Schonauer LM.
  Source: J Reprod Med. 2000 March; 45(3): 235-9.
  http://www.ncbi.nlm.nih.gov/entrez/query.fcgi?cmd=Retrieve&db=pubmed&dopt=Abstract&list_uids=10756504

- **Ovulation induction in a woman with premature ovarian failure resulting from a partial deletion of the X chromosome long arm, 46,X,del(X)(q22).**
  Author(s): Ishizuka B, Kudo Y, Amemiya A, Ogata T.
  Source: Fertility and Sterility. 1997 November; 68(5): 931-4.
  http://www.ncbi.nlm.nih.gov/entrez/query.fcgi?cmd=Retrieve&db=pubmed&dopt=Abstract&list_uids=9389828

- **Ovulation induction in premature ovarian failure: a placebo-controlled randomized trial combining pituitary suppression with gonadotropin stimulation.**
  Author(s): van Kasteren YM, Hoek A, Schoemaker J.
  Source: Fertility and Sterility. 1995 August; 64(2): 273-8.
  http://www.ncbi.nlm.nih.gov/entrez/query.fcgi?cmd=Retrieve&db=pubmed&dopt=Abstract&list_uids=7615102

- **Ovulation induction in women with premature ovarian failure: a prospective, crossover study.**
  Author(s): Rosen GF, Stone SC, Yee B.
  Source: Fertility and Sterility. 1992 February; 57(2): 448-9.
  http://www.ncbi.nlm.nih.gov/entrez/query.fcgi?cmd=Retrieve&db=pubmed&dopt=Abstract&list_uids=1735500

- **Ovulation induction with clomiphene citrate in a women with premature ovarian failure. A case report.**
  Author(s): Davis OK, Ravnikar VA.
  Source: J Reprod Med. 1988 June; 33(6): 559-62.
  http://www.ncbi.nlm.nih.gov/entrez/query.fcgi?cmd=Retrieve&db=pubmed&dopt=Abstract&list_uids=3404519

- **Persistent pregnanediol glucuronide secretion after gonadotrophin suppression indicates adrenal source of progesterone in premature ovarian failure.**
  Author(s): Sachdev R, Von Hagen S, Kamnani A, Santoro N.
  Source: Human Reproduction (Oxford, England). 1998 August; 13(8): 2061-3.
  http://www.ncbi.nlm.nih.gov/entrez/query.fcgi?cmd=Retrieve&db=pubmed&dopt=Abstract&list_uids=9756268

- **Physical mapping of nine Xq translocation breakpoints and identification of XPNPEP2 as a premature ovarian failure candidate gene.**
  Author(s): Prueitt RL, Ross JL, Zinn AR.
  Source: Cytogenetics and Cell Genetics. 2000; 89(1-2): 44-50.
  http://www.ncbi.nlm.nih.gov/entrez/query.fcgi?cmd=Retrieve&db=pubmed&dopt=Abstract&list_uids=10894934

- **Postmenopausal pregnancy: is it due to premature ovarian failure, resistant ovarian syndrome or more accurately ovarian dysfunction syndrome?**
  Author(s): Eldeen HG, Fawzi H.
  Source: Journal of Obstetrics and Gynaecology : the Journal of the Institute of Obstetrics and Gynaecology. 2003 November; 23(6): 672-3.
  http://www.ncbi.nlm.nih.gov/entrez/query.fcgi?cmd=Retrieve&db=pubmed&dopt=Abstract&list_uids=14617482

- **Pregnancies after premature ovarian failure.**
  Author(s): Alper MM, Jolly EE, Garner PR.
  Source: Obstetrics and Gynecology. 1986 March; 67(3 Suppl): 59S-62S.
  http://www.ncbi.nlm.nih.gov/entrez/query.fcgi?cmd=Retrieve&db=pubmed&dopt=Abstract&list_uids=3080719

- **Pregnancies established by gamete intrafallopian transfer and pronuclear-stage transfer in patients with premature ovarian failure using donated oocytes and low-dose oral micronized estradiol and progesterone.**
  Author(s): Olar TT, Dickey RP, Curole DN, Taylor SN.
  Source: J in Vitro Fert Embryo Transf. 1989 June; 6(3): 160-3.
  http://www.ncbi.nlm.nih.gov/entrez/query.fcgi?cmd=Retrieve&db=pubmed&dopt=Abstract&list_uids=2794733

- **Pregnancies in patients with premature ovarian failure.**
  Author(s): Gucer F, Urdl W, Pieber D, Arikan MG, Giuliani A, Auner H.
  Source: Clin Exp Obstet Gynecol. 1997; 24(3): 130-2.
  http://www.ncbi.nlm.nih.gov/entrez/query.fcgi?cmd=Retrieve&db=pubmed&dopt=Abstract&list_uids=9478295

- **Pregnancy after corticosteroid administration in premature ovarian failure (polyglandular endocrinopathy syndrome).**
  Author(s): Cowchock FS, McCabe JL, Montgomery BB.
  Source: American Journal of Obstetrics and Gynecology. 1988 January; 158(1): 118-9.
  http://www.ncbi.nlm.nih.gov/entrez/query.fcgi?cmd=Retrieve&db=pubmed&dopt=Abstract&list_uids=3337157

- **Pregnancy following in vitro fertilisation of an anonymously donated oocyte in a patient with premature ovarian failure.**
  Author(s): Cooper TK, Traub AI, Robinson SY, Thompson W.
  Source: Ulster Med J. 1989 October; 58(2): 182-6. No Abstract Available.
  http://www.ncbi.nlm.nih.gov/entrez/query.fcgi?cmd=Retrieve&db=pubmed&dopt=Abstract&list_uids=2603272

- **Pregnancy following oocyte donation and tubal embryo transfer in patients with premature ovarian failure: report of two cases.**
  Author(s): Yang YS, Hwang JL, Ho HN, Kuo YS, Lien YR, Lee TY.
  Source: J Formos Med Assoc. 1991 July; 90(7): 688-92.
  http://www.ncbi.nlm.nih.gov/entrez/query.fcgi?cmd=Retrieve&db=pubmed&dopt=Abstract&list_uids=1681021

- **Pregnancy in a patient with premature ovarian failure.**
  Author(s): Gossain VV, Carella MJ, Rovner DR.
  Source: J Med. 1993; 24(6): 393-402.
  http://www.ncbi.nlm.nih.gov/entrez/query.fcgi?cmd=Retrieve&db=pubmed&dopt=Abstract&list_uids=8182352

- **Pregnancy in a premature ovarian failure patient with donated oocytes from a 40-year-old sibling: a case report.**
  Author(s): De Silva M, Conley FA, Lee CS.
  Source: J in Vitro Fert Embryo Transf. 1991 August; 8(4): 235-6. No Abstract Available.
  http://www.ncbi.nlm.nih.gov/entrez/query.fcgi?cmd=Retrieve&db=pubmed&dopt=Abstract&list_uids=1753172

- **Pregnancy in a woman with premature ovarian failure.**
  Author(s): Finer N, Fogelman I, Bottazzo G.
  Source: Postgraduate Medical Journal. 1985 December; 61(722): 1079-80.
  http://www.ncbi.nlm.nih.gov/entrez/query.fcgi?cmd=Retrieve&db=pubmed&dopt=Abstract&list_uids=4095053

- **Pregnancy in premature ovarian failure after therapy with oral contraceptives despite resistance to previous human menopausal gonadotropin therapy.**
  Author(s): Check JH, Chase JS, Spence M.
  Source: American Journal of Obstetrics and Gynecology. 1989 January; 160(1): 114-5.
  http://www.ncbi.nlm.nih.gov/entrez/query.fcgi?cmd=Retrieve&db=pubmed&dopt=Abstract&list_uids=2492146

- **Pregnancy in premature ovarian failure: a possible role of estrogen plus progesterone treatment.**
  Author(s): Zargar AH, Salahuddin M, Wani AI, Bashir MI, Masoodi SR, Laway BA.
  Source: J Assoc Physicians India. 2000 February; 48(2): 213-5.
  http://www.ncbi.nlm.nih.gov/entrez/query.fcgi?cmd=Retrieve&db=pubmed&dopt=Abstract&list_uids=11229151

- **Pregnancy in women with premature ovarian failure using tubal and intrauterine transfer of cryopreserved zygotes.**
  Author(s): Abdalla HI, Baber RJ, Kirkland A, Leonard T, Studd JW.
  Source: British Journal of Obstetrics and Gynaecology. 1989 September; 96(9): 1071-5.
  http://www.ncbi.nlm.nih.gov/entrez/query.fcgi?cmd=Retrieve&db=pubmed&dopt=Abstract&list_uids=2804010

- **Pregnancy results following embryo transfer in women receiving low-dosage variable-length estrogen replacement therapy for premature ovarian failure.**
  Author(s): Leeton J, Rogers P, Cameron I, Caro C, Healy D.
  Source: J in Vitro Fert Embryo Transf. 1989 August; 6(4): 232-5.
  http://www.ncbi.nlm.nih.gov/entrez/query.fcgi?cmd=Retrieve&db=pubmed&dopt=Abstract&list_uids=2614218

- **Premature ovarian failure (POF) and fragile X premutation females: from POF to to fragile X carrier identification, from fragile X carrier diagnosis to POF association data.**
  Author(s): Uzielli ML, Guarducci S, Lapi E, Cecconi A, Ricci U, Ricotti G, Biondi C, Scarselli B, Vieri F, Scarnato P, Gori F, Sereni A.
  Source: American Journal of Medical Genetics. 1999 May 28; 84(3): 300-3.
  http://www.ncbi.nlm.nih.gov/entrez/query.fcgi?cmd=Retrieve&db=pubmed&dopt=Abstract&list_uids=10331612

- **Premature ovarian failure (POF): discordance between somatic and reproductive aging.**
  Author(s): Pal L, Santoro N.
  Source: Ageing Research Reviews. 2002 June; 1(3): 413-23. Review.
  http://www.ncbi.nlm.nih.gov/entrez/query.fcgi?cmd=Retrieve&db=pubmed&dopt=Abstract&list_uids=12067595

- **Premature ovarian failure among fragile X premutation carriers: parent-of-origin effect?**
  Author(s): Sherman SL.
  Source: American Journal of Human Genetics. 2000 July; 67(1): 11-3. Epub 2000 June 12.
  http://www.ncbi.nlm.nih.gov/entrez/query.fcgi?cmd=Retrieve&db=pubmed&dopt=Abstract&list_uids=10848491

- **Premature ovarian failure and autoimmune hypothyroidism in the absence of Addison's disease.**
  Author(s): Wolffenbuttel BH, Weber RF, Prins ME, Verschoor L.
  Source: The Netherlands Journal of Medicine. 1987 April; 30(3-4): 128-34.
  http://www.ncbi.nlm.nih.gov/entrez/query.fcgi?cmd=Retrieve&db=pubmed&dopt=Abstract&list_uids=3600897

- **Premature ovarian failure and endometrial ablation.**
  Author(s): Roberts LJ.
  Source: Br J Hosp Med. 1990 November; 44(5): 318. No Abstract Available.
  http://www.ncbi.nlm.nih.gov/entrez/query.fcgi?cmd=Retrieve&db=pubmed&dopt=Abstract&list_uids=2275991

- **Premature ovarian failure and FMR1 premutation co-segregation in a large Brazilian family.**
  Author(s): Machado-Ferreira MC, Costa-Lima MA, Boy RT, Esteves GS, Pimentel MM.
  Source: International Journal of Molecular Medicine. 2002 August; 10(2): 231-3.
  http://www.ncbi.nlm.nih.gov/entrez/query.fcgi?cmd=Retrieve&db=pubmed&dopt=Abstract&list_uids=12119565

- **Premature ovarian failure and fragile X premutation: a study on 45 women.**
  Author(s): Bussani C, Papi L, Sestini R, Baldinotti F, Bucciantini S, Bruni V, Scarselli G.
  Source: European Journal of Obstetrics, Gynecology, and Reproductive Biology. 2004 February 10; 112(2): 189-91.
  http://www.ncbi.nlm.nih.gov/entrez/query.fcgi?cmd=Retrieve&db=pubmed&dopt=Abstract&list_uids=14746957

- **Premature ovarian failure and FRAXA premutation: Positive correlation in a Brazilian survey.**
  Author(s): Machado-Ferreira Mdo C, Costa-Lima MA, Boy RT, Esteves GS, Pimentel MM.
  Source: American Journal of Medical Genetics. 2004 April 30; 126A(3): 237-40.
  http://www.ncbi.nlm.nih.gov/entrez/query.fcgi?cmd=Retrieve&db=pubmed&dopt=Abstract&list_uids=15054835

- **Premature ovarian failure and hypothyroidism associated with sicca syndrome.**
  Author(s): Ayala A, Canales ES, Karchmer S, Alarcon D, Zarate A.
  Source: Obstetrics and Gynecology. 1979 March; 53(3 Suppl): 98S-101S.
  http://www.ncbi.nlm.nih.gov/entrez/query.fcgi?cmd=Retrieve&db=pubmed&dopt=Abstract&list_uids=424141

- **Premature ovarian failure and ovarian autoimmunity.**
  Author(s): Hoek A, Schoemaker J, Drexhage HA.
  Source: Endocrine Reviews. 1997 February; 18(1): 107-34. Review.
  http://www.ncbi.nlm.nih.gov/entrez/query.fcgi?cmd=Retrieve&db=pubmed&dopt=Abstract&list_uids=9034788

- **Premature ovarian failure and ovarian dysgenesis associated with balanced and unbalanced X-6 translocations, respectively: implications for the investigation of ovarian failure.**
  Author(s): Center JR, McElduff A, Roberts CG.
  Source: The Australian & New Zealand Journal of Obstetrics & Gynaecology. 1994 May; 34(2): 185-8.
  http://www.ncbi.nlm.nih.gov/entrez/query.fcgi?cmd=Retrieve&db=pubmed&dopt=Abstract&list_uids=7980310

- **Premature ovarian failure and precocious puberty.**
  Author(s): Baer KA.
  Source: Obstetrics and Gynecology. 1977 January; 49(1 Suppl): 15-6.
  http://www.ncbi.nlm.nih.gov/entrez/query.fcgi?cmd=Retrieve&db=pubmed&dopt=Abstract&list_uids=831169

- **Premature ovarian failure and the FMR1 gene.**
  Author(s): Murray A.
  Source: Seminars in Reproductive Medicine. 2000; 18(1): 59-66. Review.
  http://www.ncbi.nlm.nih.gov/entrez/query.fcgi?cmd=Retrieve&db=pubmed&dopt=Abstract&list_uids=11299521

- **Premature ovarian failure associated with a Robertsonian translocation.**
  Author(s): Kawano Y, Narahara H, Matsui N, Miyakawa I.
  Source: Acta Obstetricia Et Gynecologica Scandinavica. 1998 April; 77(4): 467-9.
  http://www.ncbi.nlm.nih.gov/entrez/query.fcgi?cmd=Retrieve&db=pubmed&dopt=Abstract&list_uids=9598963

- **Premature ovarian failure associated with autoantibodies to the zona pellucida.**
  Author(s): Smith S, Hosid S.
  Source: Int J Fertil Menopausal Stud. 1994 November-December; 39(6): 316-9.
  http://www.ncbi.nlm.nih.gov/entrez/query.fcgi?cmd=Retrieve&db=pubmed&dopt=Abstract&list_uids=7889083

- **Premature ovarian failure associated with autoimmune polyglandular syndrome: pathophysiological mechanisms and future fertility.**
  Author(s): Kauffman RP, Castracane VD.
  Source: Journal of Women's Health (2002). 2003 June; 12(5): 513-20.
  http://www.ncbi.nlm.nih.gov/entrez/query.fcgi?cmd=Retrieve&db=pubmed&dopt=Abstract&list_uids=12869299

- **Premature ovarian failure associated with the candida endocrinopathy syndrome. Case report.**
  Author(s): Dempsey AT, De Swiet M, Dewhurst J.
  Source: British Journal of Obstetrics and Gynaecology. 1981 May; 88(5): 563-5.
  http://www.ncbi.nlm.nih.gov/entrez/query.fcgi?cmd=Retrieve&db=pubmed&dopt=Abstract&list_uids=7236560

- **Premature ovarian failure due to an unbalanced translocation on the X chromosome.**
  Author(s): Ashraf M, Jayawickrama NS, Bowen-Simpkins P.
  Source: Bjog : an International Journal of Obstetrics and Gynaecology. 2001 February; 108(2): 230-2.
  http://www.ncbi.nlm.nih.gov/entrez/query.fcgi?cmd=Retrieve&db=pubmed&dopt=Abstract&list_uids=11236128

- **Premature ovarian failure in a 15-year-old.**
  Author(s): Hung W, Maclaren NK, Kapur S, Anderson KD, August GP.
  Source: Clinical Pediatrics. 1986 January; 25(1): 40-2.
  http://www.ncbi.nlm.nih.gov/entrez/query.fcgi?cmd=Retrieve&db=pubmed&dopt=Abstract&list_uids=3943251

- **Premature ovarian failure in a 35-year-old woman with a Robertsonian translocation.**
  Author(s): Orczyk GP, Pehrson J, Leventhal JM.
  Source: Int J Fertil. 1989 May-June; 34(3): 184-7. No Abstract Available.
  http://www.ncbi.nlm.nih.gov/entrez/query.fcgi?cmd=Retrieve&db=pubmed&dopt=Abstract&list_uids=2567712

- **Premature ovarian failure in a female with proximal symphalangism and Noggin mutation.**
  Author(s): Kosaki K, Sato S, Hasegawa T, Matsuo N, Suzuki T, Ogata T.
  Source: Fertility and Sterility. 2004 April; 81(4): 1137-9.
  http://www.ncbi.nlm.nih.gov/entrez/query.fcgi?cmd=Retrieve&db=pubmed&dopt=Abstract&list_uids=15066478

- **Premature ovarian failure in a triple X female.**
  Author(s): Smith HC, Seale JP, Posen S.
  Source: J Obstet Gynaecol Br Commonw. 1974 May; 81(5): 405-9. No Abstract Available.
  http://www.ncbi.nlm.nih.gov/entrez/query.fcgi?cmd=Retrieve&db=pubmed&dopt=Abstract&list_uids=4832321

- **Premature ovarian failure in the fragile X syndrome.**
  Author(s): Sherman SL.
  Source: American Journal of Medical Genetics. 2000 Fall; 97(3): 189-94. Review.
  http://www.ncbi.nlm.nih.gov/entrez/query.fcgi?cmd=Retrieve&db=pubmed&dopt=Abstract&list_uids=11449487

- **Premature ovarian failure in women with epilepsy.**
  Author(s): Klein P, Serje A, Pezzullo JC.
  Source: Epilepsia. 2001 December; 42(12): 1584-9.
  http://www.ncbi.nlm.nih.gov/entrez/query.fcgi?cmd=Retrieve&db=pubmed&dopt=Abstract&list_uids=11879371

- **Premature ovarian failure in women with juvenile idiopathic arthritis (JIA).**
  Author(s): Packham JC, Hall MA.
  Source: Clin Exp Rheumatol. 2003 May-June; 21(3): 347-50.
  http://www.ncbi.nlm.nih.gov/entrez/query.fcgi?cmd=Retrieve&db=pubmed&dopt=Abstract&list_uids=12846055

- **Premature ovarian failure is associated with maternally and paternally inherited premutation in Brazilian families with fragile X.**
  Author(s): Vianna-Morgante AM, Costa SS.
  Source: American Journal of Human Genetics. 2000 July; 67(1): 254-5; Author Reply 256-8.
  http://www.ncbi.nlm.nih.gov/entrez/query.fcgi?cmd=Retrieve&db=pubmed&dopt=Abstract&list_uids=10848496

- **Premature ovarian failure is not premature menopause.**
  Author(s): Kalantaridou SN, Nelson LM.
  Source: Annals of the New York Academy of Sciences. 2000; 900: 393-402. Review.
  http://www.ncbi.nlm.nih.gov/entrez/query.fcgi?cmd=Retrieve&db=pubmed&dopt=Abstract&list_uids=10818427

- **Premature ovarian failure.**
  Author(s): Jewelewicz R, Schwartz M.
  Source: Bull N Y Acad Med. 1986 April; 62(3): 219-36. No Abstract Available.
  http://www.ncbi.nlm.nih.gov/entrez/query.fcgi?cmd=Retrieve&db=pubmed&dopt=Abstract&list_uids=3085756

- **Premature ovarian failure.**
  Author(s): Aiman J, Smentek C.
  Source: Obstetrics and Gynecology. 1985 July; 66(1): 9-14.
  http://www.ncbi.nlm.nih.gov/entrez/query.fcgi?cmd=Retrieve&db=pubmed&dopt=Abstract&list_uids=3925400

- **Premature ovarian failure.**
  Author(s): Markwood R, Magyar D.
  Source: J Am Osteopath Assoc. 1985 April; 85(4): 259-63. No Abstract Available.
  http://www.ncbi.nlm.nih.gov/entrez/query.fcgi?cmd=Retrieve&db=pubmed&dopt=Abstract&list_uids=4044322

- **Premature ovarian failure.**
  Author(s): Tulandi T, Kinch RA.
  Source: Obstetrical & Gynecological Survey. 1981 September; 36(9): 521-7.
  http://www.ncbi.nlm.nih.gov/entrez/query.fcgi?cmd=Retrieve&db=pubmed&dopt=Abstract&list_uids=7279334

- **Premature ovarian failure.**
  Author(s): Vaidya RA, Aloorkar SD, Rege NR, Joshi UM, Peter J, Sheth AR, Devi PK, Motashaw ND.
  Source: J Reprod Med. 1977 December; 19(6): 348-52.
  http://www.ncbi.nlm.nih.gov/entrez/query.fcgi?cmd=Retrieve&db=pubmed&dopt=Abstract&list_uids=145494

- **Premature ovarian failure.**
  Author(s): Starup J, Sele V.
  Source: Acta Obstetricia Et Gynecologica Scandinavica. 1973; 52(3): 259-68.
  http://www.ncbi.nlm.nih.gov/entrez/query.fcgi?cmd=Retrieve&db=pubmed&dopt=Abstract&list_uids=4743781

- **Premature ovarian failure.**
  Author(s): Sele V, Starup J.
  Source: Acta Obstetricia Et Gynecologica Scandinavica. Supplement. 1971; 9: Suppl 9: 24.
  http://www.ncbi.nlm.nih.gov/entrez/query.fcgi?cmd=Retrieve&db=pubmed&dopt=Abstract&list_uids=5287097

- **Premature ovarian failure.**
  Author(s): Conway GS.
  Source: British Medical Bulletin. 2000; 56(3): 643-9. Review.
  http://www.ncbi.nlm.nih.gov/entrez/query.fcgi?cmd=Retrieve&db=pubmed&dopt=Abstract&list_uids=11255551

- **Premature ovarian failure.**
  Author(s): Vegetti W, Marozzi A, Manfredini E, Testa G, Alagna F, Nicolosi A, Caliari I, Taborelli M, Tibiletti MG, Dalpra L, Crosignani PG.
  Source: Molecular and Cellular Endocrinology. 2000 March 30; 161(1-2): 53-7.
  http://www.ncbi.nlm.nih.gov/entrez/query.fcgi?cmd=Retrieve&db=pubmed&dopt=Abstract&list_uids=10773392

- **Premature ovarian failure.**
  Author(s): Falsetti L, Scalchi S, Villani MT, Bugari G.
  Source: Gynecological Endocrinology : the Official Journal of the International Society of Gynecological Endocrinology. 1999 June; 13(3): 189-95.
  http://www.ncbi.nlm.nih.gov/entrez/query.fcgi?cmd=Retrieve&db=pubmed&dopt=Abstract&list_uids=10451811

- **Premature ovarian failure.**
  Author(s): Kalantaridou SN, Davis SR, Nelson LM.
  Source: Endocrinology and Metabolism Clinics of North America. 1998 December; 27(4): 989-1006. Review.
  http://www.ncbi.nlm.nih.gov/entrez/query.fcgi?cmd=Retrieve&db=pubmed&dopt=Abstract&list_uids=9922918

- **Premature ovarian failure.**
  Author(s): Conway GS.
  Source: Current Opinion in Obstetrics & Gynecology. 1997 June; 9(3): 202-6. Review.
  http://www.ncbi.nlm.nih.gov/entrez/query.fcgi?cmd=Retrieve&db=pubmed&dopt=Abstract&list_uids=9263705

- **Premature ovarian failure.**
  Author(s): Barlow DH.
  Source: Baillieres Clin Obstet Gynaecol. 1996 September; 10(3): 361-84. Review. No Abstract Available.
  http://www.ncbi.nlm.nih.gov/entrez/query.fcgi?cmd=Retrieve&db=pubmed&dopt=Abstract&list_uids=8931900

- **Premature ovarian failure.**
  Author(s): Davis SR.
  Source: Maturitas. 1996 February; 23(1): 1-8. Review.
  http://www.ncbi.nlm.nih.gov/entrez/query.fcgi?cmd=Retrieve&db=pubmed&dopt=Abstract&list_uids=8861080

- **Premature ovarian failure.**
  Author(s): Speroff L.
  Source: Adv Endocrinol Metab. 1995; 6: 233-58. Review. No Abstract Available.
  http://www.ncbi.nlm.nih.gov/entrez/query.fcgi?cmd=Retrieve&db=pubmed&dopt=Abstract&list_uids=7671098

- **Premature ovarian failure.**
  Author(s): Nelson LM, Merriam GR.
  Source: American Journal of Obstetrics and Gynecology. 1990 March; 162(3): 874-6.
  http://www.ncbi.nlm.nih.gov/entrez/query.fcgi?cmd=Retrieve&db=pubmed&dopt=Abstract&list_uids=2316604

- **Premature ovarian failure. Current concepts.**
  Author(s): Alper MM, Garner PR, Seibel MM.
  Source: J Reprod Med. 1986 August; 31(8): 699-708. Review.
  http://www.ncbi.nlm.nih.gov/entrez/query.fcgi?cmd=Retrieve&db=pubmed&dopt=Abstract&list_uids=3534255

- **Premature ovarian failure. I: The association with autoimmunity.**
  Author(s): Mignot MH, Schoemaker J, Kleingeld M, Rao BR, Drexhage HA.
  Source: European Journal of Obstetrics, Gynecology, and Reproductive Biology. 1989 January; 30(1): 59-66.
  http://www.ncbi.nlm.nih.gov/entrez/query.fcgi?cmd=Retrieve&db=pubmed&dopt=Abstract&list_uids=2647538

- **Premature ovarian failure. II: Considerations of cellular immunity defects.**
  Author(s): Mignot MH, Drexhage HA, Kleingeld M, Van de Plassche-Boers EM, Rao BR, Schoemaker J.
  Source: European Journal of Obstetrics, Gynecology, and Reproductive Biology. 1989 January; 30(1): 67-72.
  http://www.ncbi.nlm.nih.gov/entrez/query.fcgi?cmd=Retrieve&db=pubmed&dopt=Abstract&list_uids=2647539

- **Premature ovarian failure. Report of seven cases.**
  Author(s): Emperaire JC, Audebert A, Greenblatt RB.
  Source: American Journal of Obstetrics and Gynecology. 1970 October 1; 108(3): 445-9.
  http://www.ncbi.nlm.nih.gov/entrez/query.fcgi?cmd=Retrieve&db=pubmed&dopt=Abstract&list_uids=5484603

- **Premature ovarian failure: a clinical, histological and cytogenetic study.**
  Author(s): Tanaka S, Mizunuma M, Watanabe H, Hata H, Shimoya Y, Hashimoto M.
  Source: Asia Oceania J Obstet Gynaecol. 1988 September; 14(3): 293-300. No Abstract Available.
  http://www.ncbi.nlm.nih.gov/entrez/query.fcgi?cmd=Retrieve&db=pubmed&dopt=Abstract&list_uids=3178575

- **Premature ovarian failure: a search for circulating factors against gonadotropin receptors.**
  Author(s): Tang VW, Faiman C.
  Source: American Journal of Obstetrics and Gynecology. 1983 August 1; 146(7): 816-21.
  http://www.ncbi.nlm.nih.gov/entrez/query.fcgi?cmd=Retrieve&db=pubmed&dopt=Abstract&list_uids=6307054

- **Premature ovarian failure: a systematic review on therapeutic interventions to restore ovarian function and achieve pregnancy.**
  Author(s): van Kasteren YM, Schoemaker J.
  Source: Human Reproduction Update. 1999 September-October; 5(5): 483-92. Review.
  http://www.ncbi.nlm.nih.gov/entrez/query.fcgi?cmd=Retrieve&db=pubmed&dopt=Abstract&list_uids=10582785

- **Premature ovarian failure: an update.**
  Author(s): Anasti JN.
  Source: Fertility and Sterility. 1998 July; 70(1): 1-15. Review.
  http://www.ncbi.nlm.nih.gov/entrez/query.fcgi?cmd=Retrieve&db=pubmed&dopt=Abstract&list_uids=9660412

- **Premature ovarian failure: autoimmunity and natural history.**
  Author(s): Betterle C, Rossi A, Dalla Pria S, Artifoni A, Pedini B, Gavasso S, Caretto A.
  Source: Clinical Endocrinology. 1993 July; 39(1): 35-43.
  http://www.ncbi.nlm.nih.gov/entrez/query.fcgi?cmd=Retrieve&db=pubmed&dopt=Abstract&list_uids=8348706

- **Premature ovarian failure: etiology and prospects.**
  Author(s): Laml T, Schulz-Lobmeyr I, Obruca A, Huber JC, Hartmann BW.
  Source: Gynecological Endocrinology : the Official Journal of the International Society of Gynecological Endocrinology. 2000 August; 14(4): 292-302. Review.
  http://www.ncbi.nlm.nih.gov/entrez/query.fcgi?cmd=Retrieve&db=pubmed&dopt=Abstract&list_uids=11075301

- **Premature ovarian failure: evidence for the autoimmune mechanism.**
  Author(s): Coulam CB, Kempers RD, Randall RV.
  Source: Fertility and Sterility. 1981 August; 36(2): 238-40.
  http://www.ncbi.nlm.nih.gov/entrez/query.fcgi?cmd=Retrieve&db=pubmed&dopt=Abstract&list_uids=6266884

- **Premature ovarian failure: frequency and risk factors among women attending a network of menopause clinics in Italy.**
  Author(s): Progetto Menopausa Italia Study Group.
  Source: Bjog : an International Journal of Obstetrics and Gynaecology. 2003 January; 110(1): 59-63.
  http://www.ncbi.nlm.nih.gov/entrez/query.fcgi?cmd=Retrieve&db=pubmed&dopt=Abstract&list_uids=12504937

- **Premature ovarian failure: its relationship to autoimmune disease.**
  Author(s): Alper MM, Garner PR.
  Source: Obstetrics and Gynecology. 1985 July; 66(1): 27-30.
  http://www.ncbi.nlm.nih.gov/entrez/query.fcgi?cmd=Retrieve&db=pubmed&dopt=Abstract&list_uids=4011067

- **Premature ovarian failure: morphological and ultrastructural aspects.**
  Author(s): Haidar MA, Baracat EC, Simoes MJ, Focchi GR, Evencio Neto J, de Lima GR.
  Source: Sao Paulo Medical Journal = Revista Paulista De Medicina. 1994 April-June; 112(2): 534-8.
  http://www.ncbi.nlm.nih.gov/entrez/query.fcgi?cmd=Retrieve&db=pubmed&dopt=Abstract&list_uids=7610321

- **Premature ovarian failure: steroid synthesis and autoimmunity.**
  Author(s): Doldi N, Belvisi L, Bassan M, Fusi FM, Ferrari A.
  Source: Gynecological Endocrinology : the Official Journal of the International Society of Gynecological Endocrinology. 1998 February; 12(1): 23-8.
  http://www.ncbi.nlm.nih.gov/entrez/query.fcgi?cmd=Retrieve&db=pubmed&dopt=Abstract&list_uids=9526706

- **Premature ovarian failure: treatment strategies.**
  Author(s): Wheeler CA.
  Source: R I Med. 1995 May; 78(5): 130-1.
  http://www.ncbi.nlm.nih.gov/entrez/query.fcgi?cmd=Retrieve&db=pubmed&dopt=Abstract&list_uids=7606058

- **Premature ovarian failure: update.**
  Author(s): Cohen I, Speroff L.
  Source: Obstetrical & Gynecological Survey. 1991 March; 46(3): 156-62. Review.
  http://www.ncbi.nlm.nih.gov/entrez/query.fcgi?cmd=Retrieve&db=pubmed&dopt=Abstract&list_uids=2014073

- **Premature ovarian failure--the prognostic application of autoimmunity on conception after ovulation induction.**
  Author(s): Blumenfeld Z, Halachmi S, Peretz BA, Shmuel Z, Golan D, Makler A, Brandes JM.
  Source: Fertility and Sterility. 1993 April; 59(4): 750-5.
  http://www.ncbi.nlm.nih.gov/entrez/query.fcgi?cmd=Retrieve&db=pubmed&dopt=Abstract&list_uids=8458491

- **Preservation of fertility and ovarian function and minimalization of chemotherapy associated gonadotoxicity and premature ovarian failure: the role of inhibin-A and -B as markers.**
  Author(s): Blumenfeld Z.
  Source: Molecular and Cellular Endocrinology. 2002 February 22; 187(1-2): 93-105. Review.
  http://www.ncbi.nlm.nih.gov/entrez/query.fcgi?cmd=Retrieve&db=pubmed&dopt=Abstract&list_uids=11988316

- **Prevalence of circulating antibodies directed toward ovaries among women with premature ovarian failure.**
  Author(s): Coulam CB, Ryan RJ.
  Source: Am J Reprod Immunol Microbiol. 1985 September; 9(1): 23-4.
  http://www.ncbi.nlm.nih.gov/entrez/query.fcgi?cmd=Retrieve&db=pubmed&dopt=Abstract&list_uids=3931487

- **Prevalence of the triple X syndrome in phenotypically normal women with premature ovarian failure and its association with autoimmune thyroid disorders.**
  Author(s): Goswami R, Goswami D, Kabra M, Gupta N, Dubey S, Dadhwal V.
  Source: Fertility and Sterility. 2003 October; 80(4): 1052-4.
  http://www.ncbi.nlm.nih.gov/entrez/query.fcgi?cmd=Retrieve&db=pubmed&dopt=Abstract&list_uids=14556833

- **Prevalence, specificity and significance of ovarian antibodies during spontaneous premature ovarian failure.**
  Author(s): Fenichel P, Sosset C, Barbarino-Monnier P, Gobert B, Hieronimus S, Bene MC, Harter M.
  Source: Human Reproduction (Oxford, England). 1997 December; 12(12): 2623-8.
  http://www.ncbi.nlm.nih.gov/entrez/query.fcgi?cmd=Retrieve&db=pubmed&dopt=Abstract&list_uids=9455825

- **Progesterone versus dehydrogesterone as replacement therapy in women with premature ovarian failure.**
  Author(s): Pellicer A, Matallin P, Miro F, Rivera J, Bonilla-Musoles FM.
  Source: Human Reproduction (Oxford, England). 1989 October; 4(7): 777-81.
  http://www.ncbi.nlm.nih.gov/entrez/query.fcgi?cmd=Retrieve&db=pubmed&dopt=Abstract&list_uids=2606955

- **Protein S levels during the normal menstrual cycle and during estrogen therapy for premature ovarian failure.**
  Author(s): Carr ME Jr, Steingold KA, Zekert SL.
  Source: The American Journal of the Medical Sciences. 1993 October; 306(4): 212-7.
  http://www.ncbi.nlm.nih.gov/entrez/query.fcgi?cmd=Retrieve&db=pubmed&dopt=Abstract&list_uids=8213888

- **Reduced ovarian complement, premature ovarian failure, and Down syndrome.**
  Author(s): Salamanca-Gomez F, Buentello L, Salamanca-Buentello F.
  Source: American Journal of Medical Genetics. 2001 March 1; 99(2): 168-9.
  http://www.ncbi.nlm.nih.gov/entrez/query.fcgi?cmd=Retrieve&db=pubmed&dopt=Abstract&list_uids=11241483

- **Regarding recall bias in the association between idiopathic premature ovarian failure and fragile X premutation.**
  Author(s): Rychlik DF.
  Source: Human Reproduction (Oxford, England). 2000 August; 15(8): 1874-5.
  http://www.ncbi.nlm.nih.gov/entrez/query.fcgi?cmd=Retrieve&db=pubmed&dopt=Abstract&list_uids=10920120

- **Relationship between serum estradiol concentration and IGF-I, IGF-II and IGF-binding proteins in patients with premature ovarian failure on short-term estradiol therapy.**
  Author(s): Elias AN, Stone SC, Tayyanipour R, Pandian MR, Rojas FJ, Gwinup G.
  Source: Int J Fertil Menopausal Stud. 1995 July-August; 40(4): 196-201.
  http://www.ncbi.nlm.nih.gov/entrez/query.fcgi?cmd=Retrieve&db=pubmed&dopt=Abstract&list_uids=8520621

- **Research on the mechanisms of premature ovarian failure.**
  Author(s): Santoro N.
  Source: Journal of the Society for Gynecologic Investigation. 2001 January-February; 8(1 Suppl Proceedings): S10-2. Review.
  http://www.ncbi.nlm.nih.gov/entrez/query.fcgi?cmd=Retrieve&db=pubmed&dopt=Abstract&list_uids=11223362

- **Resistant ovary syndrome and premature ovarian failure in young women with galactosaemia.**
  Author(s): Fraser IS, Russell P, Greco S, Robertson DM.
  Source: Clin Reprod Fertil. 1986 April; 4(2): 133-8.
  http://www.ncbi.nlm.nih.gov/entrez/query.fcgi?cmd=Retrieve&db=pubmed&dopt=Abstract&list_uids=3091236

- **Results of tubal embryo transfer in premature ovarian failure.**
  Author(s): Rotsztejn DA, Remohi J, Weckstein LN, Ord T, Moyer DL, Balmaceda JP, Asch RH.
  Source: Fertility and Sterility. 1990 August; 54(2): 348-50.
  http://www.ncbi.nlm.nih.gov/entrez/query.fcgi?cmd=Retrieve&db=pubmed&dopt=Abstract&list_uids=2379637

- **Reversal of apparent premature ovarian failure in a patient with myasthenia gravis.**
  Author(s): Bateman BG, Nunley WC Jr, Kitchin JD 3rd.
  Source: Fertility and Sterility. 1983 January; 39(1): 108-10.
  http://www.ncbi.nlm.nih.gov/entrez/query.fcgi?cmd=Retrieve&db=pubmed&dopt=Abstract&list_uids=6293884

- **Risk factors for premature ovarian failure in females with galactosemia.**
  Author(s): Guerrero NV, Singh RH, Manatunga A, Berry GT, Steiner RD, Elsas LJ 2nd.
  Source: The Journal of Pediatrics. 2000 December; 137(6): 833-41.
  http://www.ncbi.nlm.nih.gov/entrez/query.fcgi?cmd=Retrieve&db=pubmed&dopt=Abstract&list_uids=11113841

- **Routine endocrine screening for patients with karyotypically normal spontaneous premature ovarian failure.**
  Author(s): Kim TJ, Anasti JN, Flack MR, Kimzey LM, Defensor RA, Nelson LM.
  Source: Obstetrics and Gynecology. 1997 May; 89(5 Pt 1): 777-9.
  http://www.ncbi.nlm.nih.gov/entrez/query.fcgi?cmd=Retrieve&db=pubmed&dopt=Abstract&list_uids=9166320

- **Serum concentrations of follicle stimulating hormone may predict premature ovarian failure in FRAXA premutation women.**
  Author(s): Murray A, Webb J, MacSwiney F, Shipley EL, Morton NE, Conway GS.
  Source: Human Reproduction (Oxford, England). 1999 May; 14(5): 1217-8.
  http://www.ncbi.nlm.nih.gov/entrez/query.fcgi?cmd=Retrieve&db=pubmed&dopt=Abstract&list_uids=10325264

- **Serum levels of androstenedione, testosterone and dehydroepiandrosterone sulfate in patients with premature ovarian failure to age-matched menstruating controls.**
  Author(s): Elias AN, Pandian MR, Rojas FJ.
  Source: Gynecologic and Obstetric Investigation. 1997; 43(1): 47-8.
  http://www.ncbi.nlm.nih.gov/entrez/query.fcgi?cmd=Retrieve&db=pubmed&dopt=Abstract&list_uids=9015699

- **Sex hormone levels and gonadotrophin release in premature ovarian failure.**
  Author(s): Duignan NM, Shaw RW, Glass MR, Butt WR, Edwards RL.
  Source: British Journal of Obstetrics and Gynaecology. 1978 November; 85(11): 862-7.
  http://www.ncbi.nlm.nih.gov/entrez/query.fcgi?cmd=Retrieve&db=pubmed&dopt=Abstract&list_uids=718811

- **Sisters of women with premature ovarian failure may not be ideal ovum donors.**
  Author(s): Sung L, Bustillo M, Mukherjee T, Booth G, Karstaedt A, Copperman AB.
  Source: Fertility and Sterility. 1997 May; 67(5): 912-6.
  http://www.ncbi.nlm.nih.gov/entrez/query.fcgi?cmd=Retrieve&db=pubmed&dopt=Abstract&list_uids=9130899

- **Spontaneous and pharmacologically induced remissions in patients with premature ovarian failure.**
  Author(s): Kreiner D, Droesch K, Navot D, Scott R, Rosenwaks Z.
  Source: Obstetrics and Gynecology. 1988 December; 72(6): 926-8.
  http://www.ncbi.nlm.nih.gov/entrez/query.fcgi?cmd=Retrieve&db=pubmed&dopt=Abstract&list_uids=3141855

- **Spontaneous bilateral ovarian hemorrhages as a cause of premature ovarian failure.**
  Author(s): Coulam BC, Field CS, Kempers RD.
  Source: Mayo Clinic Proceedings. 1981 December; 56(12): 762-4.
  http://www.ncbi.nlm.nih.gov/entrez/query.fcgi?cmd=Retrieve&db=pubmed&dopt=Abstract&list_uids=7311604

- **Spontaneous long-term remission in a patient with premature ovarian failure.**
  Author(s): Patel B, Haddad R, Saxena I, Gossain VV.
  Source: Endocrine Practice : Official Journal of the American College of Endocrinology and the American Association of Clinical Endocrinologists. 2003 September-October; 9(5): 380-3. Review.
  http://www.ncbi.nlm.nih.gov/entrez/query.fcgi?cmd=Retrieve&db=pubmed&dopt=Abstract&list_uids=14583420

- **Spontaneous pregnancies despite failed attempts at ovulation induction in a woman with Iatrogenic premature ovarian failure.**
  Author(s): Menashe Y, Pearlstone AC, Surrey ES.
  Source: J Reprod Med. 1996 March; 41(3): 207-10.
  http://www.ncbi.nlm.nih.gov/entrez/query.fcgi?cmd=Retrieve&db=pubmed&dopt=Abstract&list_uids=8778425

- **Spontaneous pregnancy after previous pregnancy by oocyte donation due to premature ovarian failure.**
  Author(s): Sheu BC, Ho HN, Yang YS.
  Source: Human Reproduction (Oxford, England). 1996 June; 11(6): 1359-60.
  http://www.ncbi.nlm.nih.gov/entrez/query.fcgi?cmd=Retrieve&db=pubmed&dopt=Abstract&list_uids=8671459

- **Spontaneous pregnancy in a woman with lupus and thyroiditis despite imminent premature ovarian failure.**
  Author(s): Le Thi Huong D, Gompel A, Wechsler B, Piette JC.
  Source: Annals of the Rheumatic Diseases. 2004 January; 63(1): 108-9.
  http://www.ncbi.nlm.nih.gov/entrez/query.fcgi?cmd=Retrieve&db=pubmed&dopt=Abstract&list_uids=14672906

- **Spontaneous pregnancy in patients with premature ovarian failure.**
  Author(s): Chen FP, Chang SY.
  Source: Acta Obstetricia Et Gynecologica Scandinavica. 1997 January; 76(1): 81-2.
  http://www.ncbi.nlm.nih.gov/entrez/query.fcgi?cmd=Retrieve&db=pubmed&dopt=Abstract&list_uids=9033250

- **Steroid-cell autoantibodies are preferentially expressed in women with premature ovarian failure who have adrenal autoimmunity.**
  Author(s): Falorni A, Laureti S, Candeloro P, Perrino S, Coronella C, Bizzarro A, Bellastella A, Santeusanio F, De Bellis A.
  Source: Fertility and Sterility. 2002 August; 78(2): 270-9.
  http://www.ncbi.nlm.nih.gov/entrez/query.fcgi?cmd=Retrieve&db=pubmed&dopt=Abstract&list_uids=12137862

- **Studies of FRAXA and FRAXE in women with premature ovarian failure.**
  Author(s): Murray A, Webb J, Grimley S, Conway G, Jacobs P.
  Source: Journal of Medical Genetics. 1998 August; 35(8): 637-40.
  http://www.ncbi.nlm.nih.gov/entrez/query.fcgi?cmd=Retrieve&db=pubmed&dopt=Abstract&list_uids=9719368

- **Success in inducing ovulation In a case of premature ovarian failure using growth hormone-releasing hormone.**
  Author(s): Busacca M, Fusi FM, Brigante C, Doldi N, Vignali M.
  Source: Gynecological Endocrinology : the Official Journal of the International Society of Gynecological Endocrinology. 1996 August; 10(4): 277-9.
  http://www.ncbi.nlm.nih.gov/entrez/query.fcgi?cmd=Retrieve&db=pubmed&dopt=Abstract&list_uids=8908529

- **Success of donor oocyte in in vitro fertilization-embryo transfer in recipients with and without premature ovarian failure.**
  Author(s): Lydic ML, Liu JH, Rebar RW, Thomas MA, Cedars MI.
  Source: Fertility and Sterility. 1996 January; 65(1): 98-102.
  http://www.ncbi.nlm.nih.gov/entrez/query.fcgi?cmd=Retrieve&db=pubmed&dopt=Abstract&list_uids=8557162

- **Successful pregnancies after combined pentoxifylline-tocopherol treatment in women with premature ovarian failure who are resistant to hormone replacement therapy.**
  Author(s): Letur-Konirsch H, Delanian S.
  Source: Fertility and Sterility. 2003 February; 79(2): 439-41.
  http://www.ncbi.nlm.nih.gov/entrez/query.fcgi?cmd=Retrieve&db=pubmed&dopt=Abstract&list_uids=12568863

- **Successful pregnancy following oocyte donation in a patient with Diamond-Blackfan syndrome and premature ovarian failure.**
  Author(s): Aird IA, Biljan MM, Stevenson P, Kingsland CR.
  Source: Human Reproduction (Oxford, England). 1996 May; 11(5): 1123-5.
  http://www.ncbi.nlm.nih.gov/entrez/query.fcgi?cmd=Retrieve&db=pubmed&dopt=Abstract&list_uids=8671403

- **Successful pregnancy in a woman with premature ovarian failure.**
  Author(s): Fujii S, Ikeda S, Tachizaki T, Kagiya A, Saito Y.
  Source: Asia Oceania J Obstet Gynaecol. 1993 June; 19(2): 177-80.
  http://www.ncbi.nlm.nih.gov/entrez/query.fcgi?cmd=Retrieve&db=pubmed&dopt=Abstract&list_uids=8379866

- **Suppression of gonadotrophin secretion does not reverse premature ovarian failure.**
  Author(s): van der Weiden RM, Helmerhorst FM.
  Source: British Journal of Obstetrics and Gynaecology. 1989 July; 96(7): 881.
  http://www.ncbi.nlm.nih.gov/entrez/query.fcgi?cmd=Retrieve&db=pubmed&dopt=Abstract&list_uids=2504272

- **Suppression of gonadotrophin secretion does not reverse premature ovarian failure.**
  Author(s): Ledger WL, Thomas EJ, Browning D, Lenton EA, Cooke ID.
  Source: British Journal of Obstetrics and Gynaecology. 1989 February; 96(2): 196-9.
  http://www.ncbi.nlm.nih.gov/entrez/query.fcgi?cmd=Retrieve&db=pubmed&dopt=Abstract&list_uids=2522795

- **Surface ultrastructure of uterine epithelial cells in women with premature ovarian failure following steroid hormone replacement.**
  Author(s): Murphy CR, Rogers PA, Leeton J, Hosie M, Beaton L, Macpherson A.
  Source: Acta Anatomica. 1987; 130(4): 348-50.
  http://www.ncbi.nlm.nih.gov/entrez/query.fcgi?cmd=Retrieve&db=pubmed&dopt=Abstract&list_uids=3434190

- **Telomerase activity in normal ovaries and premature ovarian failure.**
  Author(s): Kinugawa C, Murakami T, Okamura K, Yajima A.
  Source: The Tohoku Journal of Experimental Medicine. 2000 March; 190(3): 231-8.
  http://www.ncbi.nlm.nih.gov/entrez/query.fcgi?cmd=Retrieve&db=pubmed&dopt=Abstract&list_uids=10778807

- **Testosterone and androstenedione in premature ovarian failure pregnancies: evidence for an ovarian source of androgens in early pregnancy.**
  Author(s): Castracane VD, Asch RH.
  Source: Human Reproduction (Oxford, England). 1995 March; 10(3): 677-80.
  http://www.ncbi.nlm.nih.gov/entrez/query.fcgi?cmd=Retrieve&db=pubmed&dopt=Abstract&list_uids=7782452

- **The effect of genetic differences and ovarian failure: intact cognitive function in adult women with premature ovarian failure versus turner syndrome.**
  Author(s): Ross JL, Stefanatos GA, Kushner H, Bondy C, Nelson L, Zinn A, Roeltgen D.
  Source: The Journal of Clinical Endocrinology and Metabolism. 2004 April; 89(4): 1817-22.
  http://www.ncbi.nlm.nih.gov/entrez/query.fcgi?cmd=Retrieve&db=pubmed&dopt=Abstract&list_uids=15070950

- **The effect of gonadotropin suppression on the induction of ovulation in premature ovarian failure patients.**
  Author(s): Surrey ES, Cedars MI.
  Source: Fertility and Sterility. 1989 July; 52(1): 36-41.
  http://www.ncbi.nlm.nih.gov/entrez/query.fcgi?cmd=Retrieve&db=pubmed&dopt=Abstract&list_uids=2526032

- **The follicle-stimulating hormone receptor gene is polymorphic in premature ovarian failure and normal controls.**
  Author(s): Whitney EA, Layman LC, Chan PJ, Lee A, Peak DB, McDonough PG.
  Source: Fertility and Sterility. 1995 September; 64(3): 518-24.
  http://www.ncbi.nlm.nih.gov/entrez/query.fcgi?cmd=Retrieve&db=pubmed&dopt=Abstract&list_uids=7641904

- **The lived experience of premature ovarian failure.**
  Author(s): Orshan SA, Furniss KK, Forst C, Santoro N.
  Source: Journal of Obstetric, Gynecologic, and Neonatal Nursing : Jognn / Naacog. 2001 March-April; 30(2): 202-8.
  http://www.ncbi.nlm.nih.gov/entrez/query.fcgi?cmd=Retrieve&db=pubmed&dopt=Abstract&list_uids=11308110

- The pathology of premature ovarian failure.
  Author(s): Fox H.
  Source: The Journal of Pathology. 1992 August; 167(4): 357-63. Review.
  http://www.ncbi.nlm.nih.gov/entrez/query.fcgi?cmd=Retrieve&db=pubmed&dopt=Abstract&list_uids=1403356

- **The use of human recombinant gonadotropin receptors to search for immunoglobulin G-mediated premature ovarian failure.**
  Author(s): Anasti JN, Flack MR, Froehlich J, Nelson LM.
  Source: The Journal of Clinical Endocrinology and Metabolism. 1995 March; 80(3): 824-8.
  http://www.ncbi.nlm.nih.gov/entrez/query.fcgi?cmd=Retrieve&db=pubmed&dopt=Abstract&list_uids=7883837

- **The variation of endometrial response to a standard hormone replacement therapy in women with premature ovarian failure. An ultrasonographic and histological study.**
  Author(s): Li TC, Dockery P, Ramsewak SS, Klentzeris L, Lenton EA, Cooke ID.
  Source: British Journal of Obstetrics and Gynaecology. 1991 July; 98(7): 656-61.
  http://www.ncbi.nlm.nih.gov/entrez/query.fcgi?cmd=Retrieve&db=pubmed&dopt=Abstract&list_uids=1883788

- Treatment concepts for premature ovarian failure.
  Author(s): van Kasteren Y.
  Source: Journal of the Society for Gynecologic Investigation. 2001 January-February; 8(1 Suppl Proceedings): S58-9. Review.
  http://www.ncbi.nlm.nih.gov/entrez/query.fcgi?cmd=Retrieve&db=pubmed&dopt=Abstract&list_uids=11223376

- **Treatment of autoimmune premature ovarian failure.**
  Author(s): Kalantaridou SN, Braddock DT, Patronas NJ, Nelson LM.
  Source: Human Reproduction (Oxford, England). 1999 July; 14(7): 1777-82.
  http://www.ncbi.nlm.nih.gov/entrez/query.fcgi?cmd=Retrieve&db=pubmed&dopt=Abstract&list_uids=10402388

- **Triplet pregnancy in premature ovarian failure after oocyte donation and in vitro fertilization: a case report and review of literature.**
  Author(s): Chen MJ, Chiue FL, Ho ES.
  Source: Zhonghua Yi Xue Za Zhi (Taipei). 1993 April; 51(4): 304-8. Review.
  http://www.ncbi.nlm.nih.gov/entrez/query.fcgi?cmd=Retrieve&db=pubmed&dopt=Abstract&list_uids=8481851

- **Triple-X syndrome and premature ovarian failure.**
  Author(s): Villanueva AL, Rebar RW.
  Source: Obstetrics and Gynecology. 1983 September; 62(3 Suppl): 70S-73S.
  http://www.ncbi.nlm.nih.gov/entrez/query.fcgi?cmd=Retrieve&db=pubmed&dopt=Abstract&list_uids=6410314

- **True 47,XXX in a patient with premature ovarian failure: the first reported case in Thailand.**
  Author(s): Tungphaisal S, Jinorose U.
  Source: J Med Assoc Thai. 1992 November; 75(11): 661-5.
  http://www.ncbi.nlm.nih.gov/entrez/query.fcgi?cmd=Retrieve&db=pubmed&dopt=Abstract&list_uids=1307391

- **Twin gestation two years after the diagnosis of premature ovarian failure in a woman on hormone replacement therapy. A case report.**
  Author(s): Fernandes AM, Arruda Mde S, Bedone AJ.
  Source: J Reprod Med. 2002 June; 47(6): 504-6.
  http://www.ncbi.nlm.nih.gov/entrez/query.fcgi?cmd=Retrieve&db=pubmed&dopt=Abstract&list_uids=12092022

- **Twin pregnancy in premature ovarian failure after estrogen treatment: a case report.**
  Author(s): Tang L, Sawers RS.
  Source: American Journal of Obstetrics and Gynecology. 1989 July; 161(1): 172-3.
  http://www.ncbi.nlm.nih.gov/entrez/query.fcgi?cmd=Retrieve&db=pubmed&dopt=Abstract&list_uids=2502014

- **Twinning and premature ovarian failure in premutation fragile X carriers.**
  Author(s): Vianna-Morgante AM.
  Source: American Journal of Medical Genetics. 1999 April 2; 83(4): 326.
  http://www.ncbi.nlm.nih.gov/entrez/query.fcgi?cmd=Retrieve&db=pubmed&dopt=Abstract&list_uids=10208171

- **Unusual premature ovarian failure with hypogonadotropic hyperprolactinemia and 46, XX, 13ph+.**
  Author(s): Ito M, Tamaya T.
  Source: J Med. 1999; 30(1-2): 13-7.
  http://www.ncbi.nlm.nih.gov/entrez/query.fcgi?cmd=Retrieve&db=pubmed&dopt=Abstract&list_uids=10515236

- **Urodynamic changes following hormonal replacement therapy in women with premature ovarian failure.**
  Author(s): Karram MM, Yeko TR, Sauer MV, Bhatia NN.
  Source: Obstetrics and Gynecology. 1989 August; 74(2): 208-11.
  http://www.ncbi.nlm.nih.gov/entrez/query.fcgi?cmd=Retrieve&db=pubmed&dopt=Abstract&list_uids=2546111

- **Usefulness of serial measurements of serum follicle stimulating hormone, luteinizing hormone and estradiol in patients with premature ovarian failure.**
  Author(s): Boyers SP, Luborsky JL, DeCherney AH.
  Source: Fertility and Sterility. 1988 September; 50(3): 408-12.
  http://www.ncbi.nlm.nih.gov/entrez/query.fcgi?cmd=Retrieve&db=pubmed&dopt=Abstract&list_uids=3137097

- **Uterine receptivity in women receiving steroid replacement therapy for premature ovarian failure: ultrastructural and endocrinological parameters.**
  Author(s): Rogers P, Murphy C, Cameron I, Leeton J, Hosie M, Beaton L, Macpherson A.
  Source: Human Reproduction (Oxford, England). 1989 May; 4(4): 349-54.
  http://www.ncbi.nlm.nih.gov/entrez/query.fcgi?cmd=Retrieve&db=pubmed&dopt=Abstract&list_uids=2745666

- **Viable pregnancy in a woman with premature ovarian failure treated with gonadotropin suppression and human menopausal gonadotropin stimulation. A case report.**
  Author(s): Check JH, Nowroozi K, Nazari A.
  Source: J Reprod Med. 1991 March; 36(3): 195-7.
  http://www.ncbi.nlm.nih.gov/entrez/query.fcgi?cmd=Retrieve&db=pubmed&dopt=Abstract&list_uids=1903165

- **X chromosome defects and premature ovarian failure.**
  Author(s): Shelling AN.
  Source: Aust N Z J Med. 2000 February; 30(1): 5-7. No Abstract Available.
  http://www.ncbi.nlm.nih.gov/entrez/query.fcgi?cmd=Retrieve&db=pubmed&dopt=Abstract&list_uids=10800870

- **X chromosome genes and premature ovarian failure.**
  Author(s): Bione S, Toniolo D.
  Source: Seminars in Reproductive Medicine. 2000; 18(1): 51-7. Review.
  http://www.ncbi.nlm.nih.gov/entrez/query.fcgi?cmd=Retrieve&db=pubmed&dopt=Abstract&list_uids=11299520

- **X chromosome mosaicism in patients with recurrent abortion or premature ovarian failure.**
  Author(s): Wu RC, Kuo PL, Lin SJ, Liu CH, Tzeng CC.
  Source: J Formos Med Assoc. 1993 November; 92(11): 953-6.
  http://www.ncbi.nlm.nih.gov/entrez/query.fcgi?cmd=Retrieve&db=pubmed&dopt=Abstract&list_uids=7910065

- **X/autosomal translocations in the Xq critical region associated with premature ovarian failure fall within and outside genes.**
  Author(s): Mumm S, Herrera L, Waeltz PW, Scardovi A, Nagaraja R, Esposito T, Schlessinger D, Rocchi M, Forabosco A.
  Source: Genomics. 2001 August; 76(1-3): 30-6.
  http://www.ncbi.nlm.nih.gov/entrez/query.fcgi?cmd=Retrieve&db=pubmed&dopt=Abstract&list_uids=11560122

- **X-chromosome abnormalities in women with premature ovarian failure.**
  Author(s): Devi A, Benn PA.
  Source: J Reprod Med. 1999 April; 44(4): 321-4.
  http://www.ncbi.nlm.nih.gov/entrez/query.fcgi?cmd=Retrieve&db=pubmed&dopt=Abstract&list_uids=10319299

CHAPTER 2. ALTERNATIVE MEDICINE AND PREMATURE OVARIAN FAILURE

Overview

In this chapter, we will begin by introducing you to official information sources on complementary and alternative medicine (CAM) relating to premature ovarian failure. At the conclusion of this chapter, we will provide additional sources.

National Center for Complementary and Alternative Medicine

The National Center for Complementary and Alternative Medicine (NCCAM) of the National Institutes of Health (http://nccam.nih.gov/) has created a link to the National Library of Medicine's databases to facilitate research for articles that specifically relate to premature ovarian failure and complementary medicine. To search the database, go to the following Web site: **http://www.nlm.nih.gov/nccam/camonpubmed.html**. Select "CAM on PubMed." Enter "premature ovarian failure" (or synonyms) into the search box. Click "Go." The following references provide information on particular aspects of complementary and alternative medicine that are related to premature ovarian failure:

- **Age at menopause in women with type 2 diabetes mellitus.**
  Author(s): Lopez-Lopez R, Huerta R, Malacara JM.
  Source: Menopause (New York, N.Y.). 1999 Summer; 6(2): 174-8.
  http://www.ncbi.nlm.nih.gov/entrez/query.fcgi?cmd=Retrieve&db=pubmed&dopt=Abstract&list_uids=10374226

- **Climacteric: concept, consequence and care.**
  Author(s): Taechakraichana N, Jaisamrarn U, Panyakhamlerd K, Chaikittisilpa S, Limpaphayom KK.
  Source: J Med Assoc Thai. 2002 June; 85 Suppl 1: S1-15. Review.
  http://www.ncbi.nlm.nih.gov/entrez/query.fcgi?cmd=Retrieve&db=pubmed&dopt=Abstract&list_uids=12188398

- **Effects of aging and estradiol supplementation on GH axis dynamics in women.**
  Author(s): Lieman HJ, Adel TE, Forst C, von Hagen S, Santoro N.

Source: The Journal of Clinical Endocrinology and Metabolism. 2001 August; 86(8): 3918-23.
http://www.ncbi.nlm.nih.gov/entrez/query.fcgi?cmd=Retrieve&db=pubmed&dopt=Abstract&list_uids=11502833

- **Gonadal function following chemotherapy for childhood Hodgkin's disease.**
  Author(s): Mackie EJ, Radford M, Shalet SM.
  Source: Medical and Pediatric Oncology. 1996 August; 27(2): 74-8.
  http://www.ncbi.nlm.nih.gov/entrez/query.fcgi?cmd=Retrieve&db=pubmed&dopt=Abstract&list_uids=8649323

- **Gonadal function following chemotherapy for Hodgkin's disease: a comparative study of MVPP and a seven-drug hybrid regimen.**
  Author(s): Clark ST, Radford JA, Crowther D, Swindell R, Shalet SM.
  Source: Journal of Clinical Oncology : Official Journal of the American Society of Clinical Oncology. 1995 January; 13(1): 134-9.
  http://www.ncbi.nlm.nih.gov/entrez/query.fcgi?cmd=Retrieve&db=pubmed&dopt=Abstract&list_uids=7799013

- **Induction of ovarian function by using short-term human menopausal gonadotrophin in patients with ovarian failure following cytotoxic chemotherapy for haematological malignancy.**
  Author(s): Chatterjee R, Mills W, Katz M, McGarrigle HH, Goldstone AH.
  Source: Leukemia & Lymphoma. 1993 July; 10(4-5): 383-6.
  http://www.ncbi.nlm.nih.gov/entrez/query.fcgi?cmd=Retrieve&db=pubmed&dopt=Abstract&list_uids=7693105

- **Inhibin A concentrations in the sera of young women during and after chemotherapy for lymphoma: correlation with ovarian toxicity.**
  Author(s): Blumenfeld Z, Ritter M, Shen-Orr Z, Shariki K, Ben-Shahar M, Haim N.
  Source: American Journal of Reproductive Immunology (New York, N.Y. : 1989). 1998 January; 39(1): 33-40.
  http://www.ncbi.nlm.nih.gov/entrez/query.fcgi?cmd=Retrieve&db=pubmed&dopt=Abstract&list_uids=9458932

- **Long-term gonadal dysfunction and its impact on bone mineralization in patients following COPP/ABVD chemotherapy for Hodgkin's disease.**
  Author(s): Kreuser ED, Felsenberg D, Behles C, Seibt-Jung H, Mielcarek M, Diehl V, Dahmen E, Thiel E.
  Source: Annals of Oncology : Official Journal of the European Society for Medical Oncology / Esmo. 1992 September; 3 Suppl 4: 105-10.
  http://www.ncbi.nlm.nih.gov/entrez/query.fcgi?cmd=Retrieve&db=pubmed&dopt=Abstract&list_uids=1280463

- **Long-term gonadal toxicity after therapy for Hodgkin's and non-Hodgkin's lymphoma.**
  Author(s): Bokemeyer C, Schmoll HJ, van Rhee J, Kuczyk M, Schuppert F, Poliwoda H.

Source: Annals of Hematology. 1994 March; 68(3): 105-10.
http://www.ncbi.nlm.nih.gov/entrez/query.fcgi?cmd=Retrieve&db=pubmed&dopt=Abstract&list_uids=8167175

- **Nonhormonal alternatives for the management of early menopause in younger women with breast cancer.**
  Author(s): Bachmann GA.
  Source: J Natl Cancer Inst Monogr. 1994(16): 161-7. Review.
  http://www.ncbi.nlm.nih.gov/entrez/query.fcgi?cmd=Retrieve&db=pubmed&dopt=Abstract&list_uids=7999460

- **Normal pregnancy after curative multiagent chemotherapy for choriocarcinoma with brain metastases.**
  Author(s): Bakri YN, Pedersen P, Nassar M.
  Source: Acta Obstetricia Et Gynecologica Scandinavica. 1991; 70(7-8): 611-3.
  http://www.ncbi.nlm.nih.gov/entrez/query.fcgi?cmd=Retrieve&db=pubmed&dopt=Abstract&list_uids=1785279

- **Pregnancy in premature ovarian failure after therapy using Chinese herbal medicine.**
  Author(s): Chao SL, Huang LW, Yen HR.
  Source: Chang Gung Med J. 2003 June; 26(6): 449-52.
  http://www.ncbi.nlm.nih.gov/entrez/query.fcgi?cmd=Retrieve&db=pubmed&dopt=Abstract&list_uids=12956293

- **Premature ovarian failure.**
  Author(s): de Moraes-Ruehsen M, Jones GS.
  Source: Fertility and Sterility. 1967 July-August; 18(4): 440-61.
  http://www.ncbi.nlm.nih.gov/entrez/query.fcgi?cmd=Retrieve&db=pubmed&dopt=Abstract&list_uids=6028784

- **Prevention of irreversible chemotherapy-induced ovarian damage in young women with lymphoma by a gonadotrophin-releasing hormone agonist in parallel to chemotherapy.**
  Author(s): Blumenfeld Z, Avivi I, Linn S, Epelbaum R, Ben-Shahar M, Haim N.
  Source: Human Reproduction (Oxford, England). 1996 August; 11(8): 1620-6.
  http://www.ncbi.nlm.nih.gov/entrez/query.fcgi?cmd=Retrieve&db=pubmed&dopt=Abstract&list_uids=8921104

- **Reversible ovarian failure induced by a Chinese herbal medicine: lei gong teng.**
  Author(s): Edmonds SE, Montgomery JC.
  Source: Bjog : an International Journal of Obstetrics and Gynaecology. 2003 January; 110(1): 77-8.
  http://www.ncbi.nlm.nih.gov/entrez/query.fcgi?cmd=Retrieve&db=pubmed&dopt=Abstract&list_uids=12504942

- **The effect of combination chemotherapy on ovarian function in women treated for Hodgkin's disease.**
  Author(s): Whitehead E, Shalet SM, Blackledge G, Todd I, Crowther D, Beardwell CG.

Source: Cancer. 1983 September 15; 52(6): 988-93.
http://www.ncbi.nlm.nih.gov/entrez/query.fcgi?cmd=Retrieve&db=pubmed&dopt=Abstract&list_uids=6411321

- **Treatment of secondary amenorrhea with abdomen acupuncture.**
  Author(s): Han Y.
  Source: J Tradit Chin Med. 2004 March; 24(1): 42-3. No Abstract Available.
  http://www.ncbi.nlm.nih.gov/entrez/query.fcgi?cmd=Retrieve&db=pubmed&dopt=Abstract&list_uids=15119172

- **Vinblastine reduces progesterone and prostaglandin E production by rat granulosa cells in vitro.**
  Author(s): Teaff NL, Savoy-Moore RT, Subramanian MG, Ataya KM.
  Source: Reproductive Toxicology (Elmsford, N.Y.). 1990; 4(3): 209-13.
  http://www.ncbi.nlm.nih.gov/entrez/query.fcgi?cmd=Retrieve&db=pubmed&dopt=Abstract&list_uids=2136038

Additional Web Resources

A number of additional Web sites offer encyclopedic information covering CAM and related topics. The following is a representative sample:

- Alternative Medicine Foundation, Inc.: **http://www.herbmed.org/**
- AOL: **http://search.aol.com/cat.adp?id=169&layer=&from=subcats**
- Chinese Medicine: **http://www.newcenturynutrition.com/**
- drkoop.com®: **http://www.drkoop.com/InteractiveMedicine/IndexC.html**
- Family Village: **http://www.familyvillage.wisc.edu/med_altn.htm**
- Google: **http://directory.google.com/Top/Health/Alternative/**
- Healthnotes: **http://www.healthnotes.com/**
- MedWebPlus: **http://medwebplus.com/subject/Alternative_and_Complementary_Medicine**
- Open Directory Project: **http://dmoz.org/Health/Alternative/**
- HealthGate: **http://www.tnp.com/**
- WebMD®Health: **http://my.webmd.com/drugs_and_herbs**
- WholeHealthMD.com: **http://www.wholehealthmd.com/reflib/0,1529,00.html**
- Yahoo.com: **http://dir.yahoo.com/Health/Alternative_Medicine/**

The following is a specific Web list relating to premature ovarian failure; please note that any particular subject below may indicate either a therapeutic use, or a contraindication (potential danger), and does not reflect an official recommendation:

- **General Overview**

    Menopause
    Source: Integrative Medicine Communications; www.drkoop.com

General References

A good place to find general background information on CAM is the National Library of Medicine. It has prepared within the MEDLINEplus system an information topic page dedicated to complementary and alternative medicine. To access this page, go to the MEDLINEplus site at **http://www.nlm.nih.gov/medlineplus/alternativemedicine.html**. This Web site provides a general overview of various topics and can lead to a number of general sources.

CHAPTER 3. PATENTS ON PREMATURE OVARIAN FAILURE

Overview

Patents can be physical innovations (e.g. chemicals, pharmaceuticals, medical equipment) or processes (e.g. treatments or diagnostic procedures). The United States Patent and Trademark Office defines a patent as a grant of a property right to the inventor, issued by the Patent and Trademark Office.[4] Patents, therefore, are intellectual property. For the United States, the term of a new patent is 20 years from the date when the patent application was filed. If the inventor wishes to receive economic benefits, it is likely that the invention will become commercially available within 20 years of the initial filing. It is important to understand, therefore, that an inventor's patent does not indicate that a product or service is or will be commercially available. The patent implies only that the inventor has "the right to exclude others from making, using, offering for sale, or selling" the invention in the United States. While this relates to U.S. patents, similar rules govern foreign patents.

In this chapter, we show you how to locate information on patents and their inventors. If you find a patent that is particularly interesting to you, contact the inventor or the assignee for further information. **IMPORTANT NOTE:** When following the search strategy described below, you may discover non-medical patents that use the generic term "premature ovarian failure" (or a synonym) in their titles. To accurately reflect the results that you might find while conducting research on premature ovarian failure, we have not necessarily excluded non-medical patents in this bibliography.

Patents on Premature Ovarian Failure

By performing a patent search focusing on premature ovarian failure, you can obtain information such as the title of the invention, the names of the inventor(s), the assignee(s) or the company that owns or controls the patent, a short abstract that summarizes the patent, and a few excerpts from the description of the patent. The abstract of a patent tends to be more technical in nature, while the description is often written for the public. Full patent descriptions contain much more information than is presented here (e.g. claims, references, figures, diagrams, etc.). We will tell you how to obtain this information later in the chapter.

---

[4]Adapted from the United States Patent and Trademark Office: http://www.uspto.gov/web/offices/pac/doc/general/whatis.htm.

The following is an example of the type of information that you can expect to obtain from a patent search on premature ovarian failure:

- **Diagnosis of premature ovarian failure**

    Inventor(s): Shelling; Andrew N. (Auckland, NZ)

    Assignee(s): Auckland Uniservices Limited (Auckland, NZ)

    Patent Number: 6,787,311

    Date filed: August 15, 2001

    Abstract: Methods by which a predisposition to **Premature Ovarian failure** (POF) can be determined. In particular, methods are provided for detecting whether a female has a predisposition to POF with reference to an alteration (mutation) in the gene coding inhibin.

    Excerpt(s): This invention relates to methods by which a predispostion to **premature ovarian failure** can be detected as well as to methods of diagnosis of **premature ovarian failure**. Still further, this invention relates to methods of therapy. Premature ovarian failure (POF) is a condition causing secondary amenorrhea, hypoestrogenism, and elevated gonadotrophins in women younger than 40 years. POF will occur in 1% of women before the age of 40 years and in 0.1% or 1 in 1000 women before the age of 30 years (Coulam, Adamson et al. 1986). POF can be familial, genetically inherited, or sporadic where there has been no family history of the disorder. Even though there have been many advances into the cause of POF in the last few years, especially in the field of molecular genetics, the cause of POF in most cases remains a mystery. Most women presented with idiopathic POF have normal menstrual history, age of menarche, and fertility prior to the onset of the condition. It was once thought that POF was irreversible in all cases as in menopause, however, intermittent ovarian failure has been reported, and pregnancy can occur in approximately 10% of patients subsequent to diagnosis. The most immediate concern for women with POF is the menopausal symptoms they experience due to the decrease in circulating oestradiol coupled with the psychological implications of these symptoms. The menopausal symptoms include hot flushes, night sweats, insomnia, palpitations, headaches, incontinence, and dyspareunia as a result of vaginal dryness. The psychological implication of POF not only include those associated with menopause such as forgetfulness, poor concentration, irritability and mood swings.

    Web site: http://www.delphion.com/details?pn=US06787311__

- **Test for ovarian autoimmunity by detecting autoantibodies to CYP17**

    Inventor(s): Luborsky; Judith L. (Chicago, IL)

    Assignee(s): Rush-Presbyterian-St. Luke's Medical Center (Chicago, IL)

    Patent Number: 6,458,550

    Date filed: January 7, 2000

    Abstract: Ovarian autoimmunity is implicated in ovarian dysfunction associated with **premature ovarian failure** (POF) and unexplained infertility. A rapid, quantitative, and inexpensive method of clinical diagnosis of ovarian autoimmunity is provided. Diagnosis is provided by detection of autoantibodies that react with an ovarian antigen, 17-alpha-hydroxylase. This diagnostic method is applicable to ovarian autoimmunity unassociated with polyglandular disease.

Excerpt(s): Premature ovarian failure (POF), also know as premature menopause, is defined as the secondary loss of ovarian function before the age of 40 years. POF affects about 1.3 million women in the United States alone. Coulam et al. (1983), Luborsky et al. (1999a). Known contributing factors include irradiation, chemotherapy, and chromosomal abnormalities, although many cases of POF have an unknown origin (idiopathic POF). Evidence has accumulated that the ovary is a target of an autoimmune process in women with idiopathic POF. Evidence for an autoimmune etiology includes the frequent association of POF with other autoimmune disorders, lymphocytic infiltration of the ovaries, and ovarian autoantibodies in serum. About half of all women with POF express ovarian autoantibodies. Luborsky et al. (1999a). Ovarian autoantibodies also are detected in sera of women with unexplained infertility. Women with unexplained infertility represent about 15-20% of all infertility cases (about 2% of the population). Forti et al. (1998). Unexplained infertility is defined as the inability to conceive for at least one year, despite normal results on standard tests for reproductive function, which include semen analysis, postcoital testing, ovulation, and tubal patency. Like women with POF, about half of women with unexplained infertility express ovarian autoantibodies. POF may manifest itself initially as unexplained infertility. Farhi et al. (1997).

Web site: http://www.delphion.com/details?pn=US06458550__

Patent Applications on Premature Ovarian Failure

As of December 2000, U.S. patent applications are open to public viewing.[5] Applications are patent requests which have yet to be granted. (The process to achieve a patent can take several years.) The following patent applications have been filed since December 2000 relating to premature ovarian failure:

- **Can1 and its role in mammalian infertility**

Inventor(s): Agoulnik, Alexander I.; (Houston, TX), Bishop, Colin E.; (Houston, TX), Zhu, Qichao; (Houston, TX)

Correspondence: Fulbright & Jaworski, Llp; 1301 Mckinney; Suite 5100; Houston; TX; 77010-3095; US

Patent Application Number: 20020119929

Date filed: November 2, 2001

Abstract: The present invention is directed to a Can1 mammalian sequence. Defects in this sequence result in aberrant migration and/or proliferation of primordial germ cells during embryonic development, leading to Sertoli Cell Only syndrome in males and **Premature Ovarian Failure** in females.

Excerpt(s): The present invention is related to molecular and cellular biology, development, and reproductive biology. More specifically, the present invention is related to Can1 and its role in migration and/or proliferation of primordial germ cells during embryonic development. In human populations, infertility is a common problem affecting 10-15% of all individuals. Defects in migration and/or proliferation of the primordial germ cells during embryonic development can lead to both Sertoli Cell Only syndrome (SCOS) in males and **Premature Ovarian Failure** (POF) in females, in which

---

[5] This has been a common practice outside the United States prior to December 2000.

0.3% of all young women are affected. Premature ovarian failure (POF) in women is characterized as menopause that begins before the age of 35. Some cases of POF appear to be inherited. Pellas et al. (1991) originally isolated an insertional transgenic gcd (germ-cell deficient) mouse mutant having abnormal germ-cell development, and the gcd/gcd mouse is a useful animal model of **premature ovarian failure** in human females. The gcd mutation is recessive and results in infertility in both males and females with no other detectable abnormalities in other tissues. More specifically, the germ cells were specifically depleted as early as day 11.5 of embryonic development, while the various somatic cells were apparently unaffected. Thus, the gcd locus plays an important role in the migration/proliferation of primordial germ cells to the genital ridges of developing embryos.

Web site: http://appft1.uspto.gov/netahtml/PTO/search-bool.html

Keeping Current

In order to stay informed about patents and patent applications dealing with premature ovarian failure, you can access the U.S. Patent Office archive via the Internet at the following Web address: **http://www.uspto.gov/patft/index.html**. You will see two broad options: (1) Issued Patent, and (2) Published Applications. To see a list of issued patents, perform the following steps: Under "Issued Patents," click "Quick Search." Then, type "premature ovarian failure" (or synonyms) into the "Term 1" box. After clicking on the search button, scroll down to see the various patents which have been granted to date on premature ovarian failure.

You can also use this procedure to view pending patent applications concerning premature ovarian failure. Simply go back to **http://www.uspto.gov/patft/index.html**. Select "Quick Search" under "Published Applications." Then proceed with the steps listed above.

CHAPTER 4. BOOKS ON PREMATURE OVARIAN FAILURE

Overview

This chapter provides bibliographic book references relating to premature ovarian failure. In addition to online booksellers such as **www.amazon.com** and **www.bn.com**, excellent sources for book titles on premature ovarian failure include the Combined Health Information Database and the National Library of Medicine. Your local medical library also may have these titles available for loan.

Book Summaries: Online Booksellers

Commercial Internet-based booksellers, such as Amazon.com and Barnes&Noble.com, offer summaries which have been supplied by each title's publisher. Some summaries also include customer reviews. Your local bookseller may have access to in-house and commercial databases that index all published books (e.g. Books in Print®). **IMPORTANT NOTE:** Online booksellers typically produce search results for medical and non-medical books. When searching for "premature ovarian failure" at online booksellers' Web sites, you may discover non-medical books that use the generic term "premature ovarian failure" (or a synonym) in their titles. The following is indicative of the results you might find when searching for "premature ovarian failure" (sorted alphabetically by title; follow the hyperlink to view more details at Amazon.com):

- **21st Century Complete Medical Guide to Menopause, Premature Ovarian Failure (POV), Hormone Replacement Therapy (HRT), Estrogen Therapy: Authoritative Government Documents, Clinical References, and Practical Information for Patients and Physicians** by PM Medical Health News; ISBN: 1592488366;
  http://www.amazon.com/exec/obidos/ASIN/1592488366/icongroupinterna

APPENDICES

APPENDIX A. PHYSICIAN RESOURCES

Overview

In this chapter, we focus on databases and Internet-based guidelines and information resources created or written for a professional audience.

NIH Guidelines

Commonly referred to as "clinical" or "professional" guidelines, the National Institutes of Health publish physician guidelines for the most common diseases. Publications are available at the following by relevant Institute[6]:

- Office of the Director (OD); guidelines consolidated across agencies available at **http://www.nih.gov/health/consumer/conkey.htm**

- National Institute of General Medical Sciences (NIGMS); fact sheets available at **http://www.nigms.nih.gov/news/facts/**

- National Library of Medicine (NLM); extensive encyclopedia (A.D.A.M., Inc.) with guidelines: **http://www.nlm.nih.gov/medlineplus/healthtopics.html**

- National Cancer Institute (NCI); guidelines available at **http://www.cancer.gov/cancerinfo/list.aspx?viewid=5f35036e-5497-4d86-8c2c-714a9f7c8d25**

- National Eye Institute (NEI); guidelines available at **http://www.nei.nih.gov/order/index.htm**

- National Heart, Lung, and Blood Institute (NHLBI); guidelines available at **http://www.nhlbi.nih.gov/guidelines/index.htm**

- National Human Genome Research Institute (NHGRI); research available at **http://www.genome.gov/page.cfm?pageID=10000375**

- National Institute on Aging (NIA); guidelines available at **http://www.nia.nih.gov/health/**

---

[6] These publications are typically written by one or more of the various NIH Institutes.

- National Institute on Alcohol Abuse and Alcoholism (NIAAA); guidelines available at http://www.niaaa.nih.gov/publications/publications.htm

- National Institute of Allergy and Infectious Diseases (NIAID); guidelines available at http://www.niaid.nih.gov/publications/

- National Institute of Arthritis and Musculoskeletal and Skin Diseases (NIAMS); fact sheets and guidelines available at http://www.niams.nih.gov/hi/index.htm

- National Institute of Child Health and Human Development (NICHD); guidelines available at http://www.nichd.nih.gov/publications/pubskey.cfm

- National Institute on Deafness and Other Communication Disorders (NIDCD); fact sheets and guidelines at http://www.nidcd.nih.gov/health/

- National Institute of Dental and Craniofacial Research (NIDCR); guidelines available at http://www.nidr.nih.gov/health/

- National Institute of Diabetes and Digestive and Kidney Diseases (NIDDK); guidelines available at http://www.niddk.nih.gov/health/health.htm

- National Institute on Drug Abuse (NIDA); guidelines available at http://www.nida.nih.gov/DrugAbuse.html

- National Institute of Environmental Health Sciences (NIEHS); environmental health information available at http://www.niehs.nih.gov/external/facts.htm

- National Institute of Mental Health (NIMH); guidelines available at http://www.nimh.nih.gov/practitioners/index.cfm

- National Institute of Neurological Disorders and Stroke (NINDS); neurological disorder information pages available at http://www.ninds.nih.gov/health_and_medical/disorder_index.htm

- National Institute of Nursing Research (NINR); publications on selected illnesses at http://www.nih.gov/ninr/news-info/publications.html

- National Institute of Biomedical Imaging and Bioengineering; general information at http://grants.nih.gov/grants/becon/becon_info.htm

- Center for Information Technology (CIT); referrals to other agencies based on keyword searches available at http://kb.nih.gov/www_query_main.asp

- National Center for Complementary and Alternative Medicine (NCCAM); health information available at http://nccam.nih.gov/health/

- National Center for Research Resources (NCRR); various information directories available at http://www.ncrr.nih.gov/publications.asp

- Office of Rare Diseases; various fact sheets available at http://rarediseases.info.nih.gov/html/resources/rep_pubs.html

- Centers for Disease Control and Prevention; various fact sheets on infectious diseases available at http://www.cdc.gov/publications.htm

NIH Databases

In addition to the various Institutes of Health that publish professional guidelines, the NIH has designed a number of databases for professionals.[7] Physician-oriented resources provide a wide variety of information related to the biomedical and health sciences, both past and present. The format of these resources varies. Searchable databases, bibliographic citations, full-text articles (when available), archival collections, and images are all available. The following are referenced by the National Library of Medicine:[8]

- **Bioethics:** Access to published literature on the ethical, legal, and public policy issues surrounding healthcare and biomedical research. This information is provided in conjunction with the Kennedy Institute of Ethics located at Georgetown University, Washington, D.C.: http://www.nlm.nih.gov/databases/databases_bioethics.html

- **HIV/AIDS Resources:** Describes various links and databases dedicated to HIV/AIDS research: http://www.nlm.nih.gov/pubs/factsheets/aidsinfs.html

- **NLM Online Exhibitions:** Describes "Exhibitions in the History of Medicine": http://www.nlm.nih.gov/exhibition/exhibition.html. Additional resources for historical scholarship in medicine: http://www.nlm.nih.gov/hmd/hmd.html

- **Biotechnology Information:** Access to public databases. The National Center for Biotechnology Information conducts research in computational biology, develops software tools for analyzing genome data, and disseminates biomedical information for the better understanding of molecular processes affecting human health and disease: http://www.ncbi.nlm.nih.gov/

- **Population Information:** The National Library of Medicine provides access to worldwide coverage of population, family planning, and related health issues, including family planning technology and programs, fertility, and population law and policy: http://www.nlm.nih.gov/databases/databases_population.html

- **Cancer Information:** Access to cancer oriented databases: http://www.nlm.nih.gov/databases/databases_cancer.html

- **Profiles in Science:** Offering the archival collections of prominent twentieth-century biomedical scientists to the public through modern digital technology: http://www.profiles.nlm.nih.gov/

- **Chemical Information:** Provides links to various chemical databases and references: http://sis.nlm.nih.gov/Chem/ChemMain.html

- **Clinical Alerts:** Reports the release of findings from the NIH-funded clinical trials where such release could significantly affect morbidity and mortality: http://www.nlm.nih.gov/databases/alerts/clinical_alerts.html

- **Space Life Sciences:** Provides links and information to space-based research (including NASA): http://www.nlm.nih.gov/databases/databases_space.html

- **MEDLINE:** Bibliographic database covering the fields of medicine, nursing, dentistry, veterinary medicine, the healthcare system, and the pre-clinical sciences: http://www.nlm.nih.gov/databases/databases_medline.html

---

[7] Remember, for the general public, the National Library of Medicine recommends the databases referenced in MEDLINE*plus* (http://medlineplus.gov/ or http://www.nlm.nih.gov/medlineplus/databases.html).

[8] See http://www.nlm.nih.gov/databases/databases.html.

- **Toxicology and Environmental Health Information (TOXNET):** Databases covering toxicology and environmental health: http://sis.nlm.nih.gov/Tox/ToxMain.html
- **Visible Human Interface:** Anatomically detailed, three-dimensional representations of normal male and female human bodies:
  http://www.nlm.nih.gov/research/visible/visible_human.html

The NLM Gateway[9]

The NLM (National Library of Medicine) Gateway is a Web-based system that lets users search simultaneously in multiple retrieval systems at the U.S. National Library of Medicine (NLM). It allows users of NLM services to initiate searches from one Web interface, providing one-stop searching for many of NLM's information resources or databases.[10] To use the NLM Gateway, simply go to the search site at **http://gateway.nlm.nih.gov/gw/Cmd**. Type "premature ovarian failure" (or synonyms) into the search box and click "Search." The results will be presented in a tabular form, indicating the number of references in each database category.

Results Summary

Category	Items Found
Journal Articles	993
Books / Periodicals / Audio Visual	9
Consumer Health	957
Meeting Abstracts	1
Other Collections	50
Total	2010

HSTAT[11]

HSTAT is a free, Web-based resource that provides access to full-text documents used in healthcare decision-making.[12] These documents include clinical practice guidelines, quick-reference guides for clinicians, consumer health brochures, evidence reports and technology assessments from the Agency for Healthcare Research and Quality (AHRQ), as well as AHRQ's Put Prevention Into Practice.[13] Simply search by "premature ovarian failure" (or synonyms) at the following Web site: **http://text.nlm.nih.gov**.

---

[9] Adapted from NLM: http://gateway.nlm.nih.gov/gw/Cmd?Overview.x.

[10] The NLM Gateway is currently being developed by the Lister Hill National Center for Biomedical Communications (LHNCBC) at the National Library of Medicine (NLM) of the National Institutes of Health (NIH).

[11] Adapted from HSTAT: http://www.nlm.nih.gov/pubs/factsheets/hstat.html.

[12] The HSTAT URL is http://hstat.nlm.nih.gov/.

[13] Other important documents in HSTAT include: the National Institutes of Health (NIH) Consensus Conference Reports and Technology Assessment Reports; the HIV/AIDS Treatment Information Service (ATIS) resource documents; the Substance Abuse and Mental Health Services Administration's Center for Substance Abuse Treatment (SAMHSA/CSAT) Treatment Improvement Protocols (TIP) and Center for Substance Abuse Prevention (SAMHSA/CSAP) Prevention Enhancement Protocols System (PEPS); the Public Health Service (PHS) Preventive Services Task Force's *Guide to Clinical Preventive Services*; the independent, nonfederal Task Force on Community Services' *Guide to Community Preventive Services*; and the Health Technology Advisory Committee (HTAC) of the Minnesota Health Care Commission (MHCC) health technology evaluations.

Coffee Break: Tutorials for Biologists[14]

Coffee Break is a general healthcare site that takes a scientific view of the news and covers recent breakthroughs in biology that may one day assist physicians in developing treatments. Here you will find a collection of short reports on recent biological discoveries. Each report incorporates interactive tutorials that demonstrate how bioinformatics tools are used as a part of the research process. Currently, all Coffee Breaks are written by NCBI staff.[15] Each report is about 400 words and is usually based on a discovery reported in one or more articles from recently published, peer-reviewed literature.[16] This site has new articles every few weeks, so it can be considered an online magazine of sorts. It is intended for general background information. You can access the Coffee Break Web site at the following hyperlink: **http://www.ncbi.nlm.nih.gov/Coffeebreak/**.

Other Commercial Databases

In addition to resources maintained by official agencies, other databases exist that are commercial ventures addressing medical professionals. Here are some examples that may interest you:

- **CliniWeb International:** Index and table of contents to selected clinical information on the Internet; see **http://www.ohsu.edu/cliniweb/**.

- **Medical World Search:** Searches full text from thousands of selected medical sites on the Internet; see **http://www.mwsearch.com/**.

---

[14] Adapted from **http://www.ncbi.nlm.nih.gov/Coffeebreak/Archive/FAQ.html**.

[15] The figure that accompanies each article is frequently supplied by an expert external to NCBI, in which case the source of the figure is cited. The result is an interactive tutorial that tells a biological story.

[16] After a brief introduction that sets the work described into a broader context, the report focuses on how a molecular understanding can provide explanations of observed biology and lead to therapies for diseases. Each vignette is accompanied by a figure and hypertext links that lead to a series of pages that interactively show how NCBI tools and resources are used in the research process.

APPENDIX B. PATIENT RESOURCES

Overview

Official agencies, as well as federally funded institutions supported by national grants, frequently publish a variety of guidelines written with the patient in mind. These are typically called "Fact Sheets" or "Guidelines." They can take the form of a brochure, information kit, pamphlet, or flyer. Often they are only a few pages in length. Since new guidelines on premature ovarian failure can appear at any moment and be published by a number of sources, the best approach to finding guidelines is to systematically scan the Internet-based services that post them.

Patient Guideline Sources

The remainder of this chapter directs you to sources which either publish or can help you find additional guidelines on topics related to premature ovarian failure. Due to space limitations, these sources are listed in a concise manner. Do not hesitate to consult the following sources by either using the Internet hyperlink provided, or, in cases where the contact information is provided, contacting the publisher or author directly.

The National Institutes of Health

The NIH gateway to patients is located at **http://health.nih.gov/**. From this site, you can search across various sources and institutes, a number of which are summarized below.

Topic Pages: MEDLINEplus

The National Library of Medicine has created a vast and patient-oriented healthcare information portal called MEDLINEplus. Within this Internet-based system are "health topic pages" which list links to available materials relevant to premature ovarian failure. To access this system, log on to **http://www.nlm.nih.gov/medlineplus/healthtopics.html**. From there you can either search using the alphabetical index or browse by broad topic areas. Recently, MEDLINEplus listed the following when searched for "premature ovarian failure":

Hormone Replacement Therapy
http://www.nlm.nih.gov/medlineplus/hormonereplacementtherapy.html

Infertility
http://www.nlm.nih.gov/medlineplus/infertility.html

Menopause
http://www.nlm.nih.gov/medlineplus/menopause.html

Premature Ovarian Failure
http://www.nlm.nih.gov/medlineplus/prematureovarianfailure.html

Within the health topic page dedicated to premature ovarian failure, the following was listed:

- Diagnosis/Symptoms

    Estrogen Tests
    Source: American Association for Clinical Chemistry
    http://www.labtestsonline.org/understanding/analytes/estrogen/test.html

    FSH (Follicle-Stimulating Hormone) Test
    Source: American Association for Clinical Chemistry
    http://www.labtestsonline.org/understanding/analytes/fsh/test.html

- From the National Institutes of Health

    Do I Have Premature Ovarian Failure?
    Source: National Institute of Child Health and Human Development
    http://www.nichd.nih.gov/publications/pubs/pof/index.htm

- Organizations

    National Institute of Child Health and Human Development
    http://www.nichd.nih.gov/

    North American Menopause Society
    http://www.menopause.org/

    Premature Ovarian Failure Support Group
    http://www.pofsupport.org/

- Research

    Disorders Associated with Infertility
    Source: National Institute of Child Health and Human Development
    http://www.nichd.nih.gov/womenshealth/infertility.cfm

- Teenagers

    Premature Ovarian Failure: A Guide for Teens
    Source: Children's Hospital Boston
    http://www.youngwomenshealth.org/pof.html

You may also choose to use the search utility provided by MEDLINEplus at the following Web address: **http://www.nlm.nih.gov/medlineplus/**. Simply type a keyword into the search box and click "Search." This utility is similar to the NIH search utility, with the exception that it only includes materials that are linked within the MEDLINEplus system (mostly patient-oriented information). It also has the disadvantage of generating unstructured results. We recommend, therefore, that you use this method only if you have a very targeted search.

The Combined Health Information Database (CHID)

CHID Online is a reference tool that maintains a database directory of thousands of journal articles and patient education guidelines on premature ovarian failure. CHID offers summaries that describe the guidelines available, including contact information and pricing. CHID's general Web site is **http://chid.nih.gov/**. To search this database, go to **http://chid.nih.gov/detail/detail.html**. In particular, you can use the advanced search options to look up pamphlets, reports, brochures, and information kits. The following was recently posted in this archive:

- **Do I have premature ovarian failure?**

    Source: Bethesda, MD: National Institute of Child Health and Human Development. 2003. 22 pp.

    Contact: Available from National Institute of Child Health and Human Development, Building 31, 2A32, MSC 2425, 31 Center Drive, Bethesda, MD 20892. Telephone: (301) 496-5133 or (800) 370-2943 / fax: (301) 496-7101 / e-mail: NICHDClearinghouse@mail.nih.gov / Web site: http://www.nichd.nih.gov. Available at no charge; also available from the Web site at no charge.

    Summary: This brochure focuses on **premature ovarian failure** (POF), a condition in which normal functioning of the ovaries stops before a woman reaches menopause. The brochure provides fast facts, offers an overview of POF and its causes, discusses the normal menstrual cycle and what happens differently in POF, explains the symptoms and treatment options, discusses how POF affects overall health, explains how POF affects fertility, and touches on current research. Information about additional resources is also included.

The NIH Search Utility

The NIH search utility allows you to search for documents on over 100 selected Web sites that comprise the NIH-WEB-SPACE. Each of these servers is "crawled" and indexed on an ongoing basis. Your search will produce a list of various documents, all of which will relate in some way to premature ovarian failure. The drawbacks of this approach are that the information is not organized by theme and that the references are often a mix of information for professionals and patients. Nevertheless, a large number of the listed Web sites provide useful background information. We can only recommend this route, therefore, for relatively rare or specific disorders, or when using highly targeted searches. To use the NIH search utility, visit the following Web page: **http://search.nih.gov/index.html**.

Additional Web Sources

A number of Web sites are available to the public that often link to government sites. These can also point you in the direction of essential information. The following is a representative sample:

- AOL: **http://search.aol.com/cat.adp?id=168&layer=&from=subcats**
- Family Village: **http://www.familyvillage.wisc.edu/specific.htm**
- Google: **http://directory.google.com/Top/Health/Conditions_and_Diseases/**
- Med Help International: **http://www.medhelp.org/HealthTopics/A.html**
- Open Directory Project: **http://dmoz.org/Health/Conditions_and_Diseases/**
- Yahoo.com: **http://dir.yahoo.com/Health/Diseases_and_Conditions/**
- WebMD®Health: **http://my.webmd.com/health_topics**

Finding Associations

There are several Internet directories that provide lists of medical associations with information on or resources relating to premature ovarian failure. By consulting all of associations listed in this chapter, you will have nearly exhausted all sources for patient associations concerned with premature ovarian failure.

The National Health Information Center (NHIC)

The National Health Information Center (NHIC) offers a free referral service to help people find organizations that provide information about premature ovarian failure. For more information, see the NHIC's Web site at **http://www.health.gov/NHIC/** or contact an information specialist by calling 1-800-336-4797.

Directory of Health Organizations

The Directory of Health Organizations, provided by the National Library of Medicine Specialized Information Services, is a comprehensive source of information on associations. The Directory of Health Organizations database can be accessed via the Internet at **http://www.sis.nlm.nih.gov/Dir/DirMain.html**. It is composed of two parts: DIRLINE and Health Hotlines.

The DIRLINE database comprises some 10,000 records of organizations, research centers, and government institutes and associations that primarily focus on health and biomedicine. To access DIRLINE directly, go to the following Web site: **http://dirline.nlm.nih.gov/**. Simply type in "premature ovarian failure" (or a synonym), and you will receive information on all relevant organizations listed in the database.

Health Hotlines directs you to toll-free numbers to over 300 organizations. You can access this database directly at **http://www.sis.nlm.nih.gov/hotlines/**. On this page, you are given the option to search by keyword or by browsing the subject list. When you have received your search results, click on the name of the organization for its description and contact information.

The Combined Health Information Database

Another comprehensive source of information on healthcare associations is the Combined Health Information Database. Using the "Detailed Search" option, you will need to limit your search to "Organizations" and "premature ovarian failure". Type the following hyperlink into your Web browser: **http://chid.nih.gov/detail/detail.html**. To find associations, use the drop boxes at the bottom of the search page where "You may refine your search by." For publication date, select "All Years." Then, select your preferred language and the format option "Organization Resource Sheet." Type "premature ovarian failure" (or synonyms) into the "For these words:" box. You should check back periodically with this database since it is updated every three months.

The National Organization for Rare Disorders, Inc.

The National Organization for Rare Disorders, Inc. has prepared a Web site that provides, at no charge, lists of associations organized by health topic. You can access this database at the following Web site: **http://www.rarediseases.org/search/orgsearch.html**. Type "premature ovarian failure" (or a synonym) into the search box, and click "Submit Query."

APPENDIX C. FINDING MEDICAL LIBRARIES

Overview

In this Appendix, we show you how to quickly find a medical library in your area.

Preparation

Your local public library and medical libraries have interlibrary loan programs with the National Library of Medicine (NLM), one of the largest medical collections in the world. According to the NLM, most of the literature in the general and historical collections of the National Library of Medicine is available on interlibrary loan to any library. If you would like to access NLM medical literature, then visit a library in your area that can request the publications for you.[17]

Finding a Local Medical Library

The quickest method to locate medical libraries is to use the Internet-based directory published by the National Network of Libraries of Medicine (NN/LM). This network includes 4626 members and affiliates that provide many services to librarians, health professionals, and the public. To find a library in your area, simply visit **http://nnlm.gov/members/adv.html** or call 1-800-338-7657.

Medical Libraries in the U.S. and Canada

In addition to the NN/LM, the National Library of Medicine (NLM) lists a number of libraries with reference facilities that are open to the public. The following is the NLM's list and includes hyperlinks to each library's Web site. These Web pages can provide information on hours of operation and other restrictions. The list below is a small sample of

---

[17] Adapted from the NLM: **http://www.nlm.nih.gov/psd/cas/interlibrary.html**.

libraries recommended by the National Library of Medicine (sorted alphabetically by name of the U.S. state or Canadian province where the library is located)[18]:

- **Alabama:** Health InfoNet of Jefferson County (Jefferson County Library Cooperative, Lister Hill Library of the Health Sciences), **http://www.uab.edu/infonet/**
- **Alabama:** Richard M. Scrushy Library (American Sports Medicine Institute)
- **Arizona:** Samaritan Regional Medical Center: The Learning Center (Samaritan Health System, Phoenix, Arizona), **http://www.samaritan.edu/library/bannerlibs.htm**
- **California:** Kris Kelly Health Information Center (St. Joseph Health System, Humboldt), **http://www.humboldt1.com/~kkhic/index.html**
- **California:** Community Health Library of Los Gatos, **http://www.healthlib.org/orgresources.html**
- **California:** Consumer Health Program and Services (CHIPS) (County of Los Angeles Public Library, Los Angeles County Harbor-UCLA Medical Center Library) - Carson, CA, **http://www.colapublib.org/services/chips.html**
- **California:** Gateway Health Library (Sutter Gould Medical Foundation)
- **California:** Health Library (Stanford University Medical Center), **http://www-med.stanford.edu/healthlibrary/**
- **California:** Patient Education Resource Center - Health Information and Resources (University of California, San Francisco), **http://sfghdean.ucsf.edu/barnett/PERC/default.asp**
- **California:** Redwood Health Library (Petaluma Health Care District), **http://www.phcd.org/rdwdlib.html**
- **California:** Los Gatos PlaneTree Health Library, **http://planetreesanjose.org/**
- **California:** Sutter Resource Library (Sutter Hospitals Foundation, Sacramento), **http://suttermedicalcenter.org/library/**
- **California:** Health Sciences Libraries (University of California, Davis), **http://www.lib.ucdavis.edu/healthsci/**
- **California:** ValleyCare Health Library & Ryan Comer Cancer Resource Center (ValleyCare Health System, Pleasanton), **http://gaelnet.stmarys-ca.edu/other.libs/gbal/east/vchl.html**
- **California:** Washington Community Health Resource Library (Fremont), **http://www.healthlibrary.org/**
- **Colorado:** William V. Gervasini Memorial Library (Exempla Healthcare), **http://www.saintjosephdenver.org/yourhealth/libraries/**
- **Connecticut:** Hartford Hospital Health Science Libraries (Hartford Hospital), **http://www.harthosp.org/library/**
- **Connecticut:** Healthnet: Connecticut Consumer Health Information Center (University of Connecticut Health Center, Lyman Maynard Stowe Library), **http://library.uchc.edu/departm/hnet/**

---

[18] Abstracted from **http://www.nlm.nih.gov/medlineplus/libraries.html**.

- **Connecticut:** Waterbury Hospital Health Center Library (Waterbury Hospital, Waterbury), http://www.waterburyhospital.com/library/consumer.shtml
- **Delaware:** Consumer Health Library (Christiana Care Health System, Eugene du Pont Preventive Medicine & Rehabilitation Institute, Wilmington), http://www.christianacare.org/health_guide/health_guide_pmri_health_info.cfm
- **Delaware:** Lewis B. Flinn Library (Delaware Academy of Medicine, Wilmington), http://www.delamed.org/chls.html
- **Georgia:** Family Resource Library (Medical College of Georgia, Augusta), http://cmc.mcg.edu/kids_families/fam_resources/fam_res_lib/frl.htm
- **Georgia:** Health Resource Center (Medical Center of Central Georgia, Macon), http://www.mccg.org/hrc/hrchome.asp
- **Hawaii:** Hawaii Medical Library: Consumer Health Information Service (Hawaii Medical Library, Honolulu), http://hml.org/CHIS/
- **Idaho:** DeArmond Consumer Health Library (Kootenai Medical Center, Coeur d'Alene), http://www.nicon.org/DeArmond/index.htm
- **Illinois:** Health Learning Center of Northwestern Memorial Hospital (Chicago), http://www.nmh.org/health_info/hlc.html
- **Illinois:** Medical Library (OSF Saint Francis Medical Center, Peoria), http://www.osfsaintfrancis.org/general/library/
- **Kentucky:** Medical Library - Services for Patients, Families, Students & the Public (Central Baptist Hospital, Lexington), http://www.centralbap.com/education/community/library.cfm
- **Kentucky:** University of Kentucky - Health Information Library (Chandler Medical Center, Lexington), http://www.mc.uky.edu/PatientEd/
- **Louisiana:** Alton Ochsner Medical Foundation Library (Alton Ochsner Medical Foundation, New Orleans), http://www.ochsner.org/library/
- **Louisiana:** Louisiana State University Health Sciences Center Medical Library-Shreveport, http://lib-sh.lsuhsc.edu/
- **Maine:** Franklin Memorial Hospital Medical Library (Franklin Memorial Hospital, Farmington), http://www.fchn.org/fmh/lib.htm
- **Maine:** Gerrish-True Health Sciences Library (Central Maine Medical Center, Lewiston), http://www.cmmc.org/library/library.html
- **Maine:** Hadley Parrot Health Science Library (Eastern Maine Healthcare, Bangor), http://www.emh.org/hll/hpl/guide.htm
- **Maine:** Maine Medical Center Library (Maine Medical Center, Portland), http://www.mmc.org/library/
- **Maine:** Parkview Hospital (Brunswick), http://www.parkviewhospital.org/
- **Maine:** Southern Maine Medical Center Health Sciences Library (Southern Maine Medical Center, Biddeford), http://www.smmc.org/services/service.php3?choice=10
- **Maine:** Stephens Memorial Hospital's Health Information Library (Western Maine Health, Norway), http://www.wmhcc.org/Library/

- **Manitoba, Canada:** Consumer & Patient Health Information Service (University of Manitoba Libraries), http://www.umanitoba.ca/libraries/units/health/reference/chis.html
- **Manitoba, Canada:** J.W. Crane Memorial Library (Deer Lodge Centre, Winnipeg), http://www.deerlodge.mb.ca/crane_library/about.asp
- **Maryland:** Health Information Center at the Wheaton Regional Library (Montgomery County, Dept. of Public Libraries, Wheaton Regional Library), http://www.mont.lib.md.us/healthinfo/hic.asp
- **Massachusetts:** Baystate Medical Center Library (Baystate Health System), http://www.baystatehealth.com/1024/
- **Massachusetts:** Boston University Medical Center Alumni Medical Library (Boston University Medical Center), http://med-libwww.bu.edu/library/lib.html
- **Massachusetts:** Lowell General Hospital Health Sciences Library (Lowell General Hospital, Lowell), http://www.lowellgeneral.org/library/HomePageLinks/WWW.htm
- **Massachusetts:** Paul E. Woodard Health Sciences Library (New England Baptist Hospital, Boston), http://www.nebh.org/health_lib.asp
- **Massachusetts:** St. Luke's Hospital Health Sciences Library (St. Luke's Hospital, Southcoast Health System, New Bedford), http://www.southcoast.org/library/
- **Massachusetts:** Treadwell Library Consumer Health Reference Center (Massachusetts General Hospital), http://www.mgh.harvard.edu/library/chrcindex.html
- **Massachusetts:** UMass HealthNet (University of Massachusetts Medical School, Worchester), http://healthnet.umassmed.edu/
- **Michigan:** Botsford General Hospital Library - Consumer Health (Botsford General Hospital, Library & Internet Services), http://www.botsfordlibrary.org/consumer.htm
- **Michigan:** Helen DeRoy Medical Library (Providence Hospital and Medical Centers), http://www.providence-hospital.org/library/
- **Michigan:** Marquette General Hospital - Consumer Health Library (Marquette General Hospital, Health Information Center), http://www.mgh.org/center.html
- **Michigan:** Patient Education Resouce Center - University of Michigan Cancer Center (University of Michigan Comprehensive Cancer Center, Ann Arbor), http://www.cancer.med.umich.edu/learn/leares.htm
- **Michigan:** Sladen Library & Center for Health Information Resources - Consumer Health Information (Detroit), http://www.henryford.com/body.cfm?id=39330
- **Montana:** Center for Health Information (St. Patrick Hospital and Health Sciences Center, Missoula)
- **National:** Consumer Health Library Directory (Medical Library Association, Consumer and Patient Health Information Section), http://caphis.mlanet.org/directory/index.html
- **National:** National Network of Libraries of Medicine (National Library of Medicine) - provides library services for health professionals in the United States who do not have access to a medical library, http://nnlm.gov/
- **National:** NN/LM List of Libraries Serving the Public (National Network of Libraries of Medicine), http://nnlm.gov/members/

- **Nevada:** Health Science Library, West Charleston Library (Las Vegas-Clark County Library District, Las Vegas), http://www.lvccld.org/special_collections/medical/index.htm
- **New Hampshire:** Dartmouth Biomedical Libraries (Dartmouth College Library, Hanover), http://www.dartmouth.edu/~biomed/resources.htmld/conshealth.htmld/
- **New Jersey:** Consumer Health Library (Rahway Hospital, Rahway), http://www.rahwayhospital.com/library.htm
- **New Jersey:** Dr. Walter Phillips Health Sciences Library (Englewood Hospital and Medical Center, Englewood), http://www.englewoodhospital.com/links/index.htm
- **New Jersey:** Meland Foundation (Englewood Hospital and Medical Center, Englewood), http://www.geocities.com/ResearchTriangle/9360/
- **New York:** Choices in Health Information (New York Public Library) - NLM Consumer Pilot Project participant, http://www.nypl.org/branch/health/links.html
- **New York:** Health Information Center (Upstate Medical University, State University of New York, Syracuse), http://www.upstate.edu/library/hic/
- **New York:** Health Sciences Library (Long Island Jewish Medical Center, New Hyde Park), http://www.lij.edu/library/library.html
- **New York:** ViaHealth Medical Library (Rochester General Hospital), http://www.nyam.org/library/
- **Ohio:** Consumer Health Library (Akron General Medical Center, Medical & Consumer Health Library), http://www.akrongeneral.org/hwlibrary.htm
- **Oklahoma:** The Health Information Center at Saint Francis Hospital (Saint Francis Health System, Tulsa), http://www.sfh-tulsa.com/services/healthinfo.asp
- **Oregon:** Planetree Health Resource Center (Mid-Columbia Medical Center, The Dalles), http://www.mcmc.net/phrc/
- **Pennsylvania:** Community Health Information Library (Milton S. Hershey Medical Center, Hershey), http://www.hmc.psu.edu/commhealth/
- **Pennsylvania:** Community Health Resource Library (Geisinger Medical Center, Danville), http://www.geisinger.edu/education/commlib.shtml
- **Pennsylvania:** HealthInfo Library (Moses Taylor Hospital, Scranton), http://www.mth.org/healthwellness.html
- **Pennsylvania:** Hopwood Library (University of Pittsburgh, Health Sciences Library System, Pittsburgh), http://www.hsls.pitt.edu/guides/chi/hopwood/index_html
- **Pennsylvania:** Koop Community Health Information Center (College of Physicians of Philadelphia), http://www.collphyphil.org/kooppg1.shtml
- **Pennsylvania:** Learning Resources Center - Medical Library (Susquehanna Health System, Williamsport), http://www.shscares.org/services/lrc/index.asp
- **Pennsylvania:** Medical Library (UPMC Health System, Pittsburgh), http://www.upmc.edu/passavant/library.htm
- **Quebec, Canada:** Medical Library (Montreal General Hospital), http://www.mghlib.mcgill.ca/

- **South Dakota:** Rapid City Regional Hospital Medical Library (Rapid City Regional Hospital), http://www.rcrh.org/Services/Library/Default.asp
- **Texas:** Houston HealthWays (Houston Academy of Medicine-Texas Medical Center Library), http://hhw.library.tmc.edu/
- **Washington:** Community Health Library (Kittitas Valley Community Hospital), http://www.kvch.com/
- **Washington:** Southwest Washington Medical Center Library (Southwest Washington Medical Center, Vancouver), http://www.swmedicalcenter.com/body.cfm?id=72

ONLINE GLOSSARIES

The Internet provides access to a number of free-to-use medical dictionaries. The National Library of Medicine has compiled the following list of online dictionaries:

- ADAM Medical Encyclopedia (A.D.A.M., Inc.), comprehensive medical reference: http://www.nlm.nih.gov/medlineplus/encyclopedia.html

- MedicineNet.com Medical Dictionary (MedicineNet, Inc.): http://www.medterms.com/Script/Main/hp.asp

- Merriam-Webster Medical Dictionary (Inteli-Health, Inc.): http://www.intelihealth.com/IH/

- Multilingual Glossary of Technical and Popular Medical Terms in Eight European Languages (European Commission) - Danish, Dutch, English, French, German, Italian, Portuguese, and Spanish: http://allserv.rug.ac.be/~rvdstich/eugloss/welcome.html

- On-line Medical Dictionary (CancerWEB): http://cancerweb.ncl.ac.uk/omd/

- Rare Diseases Terms (Office of Rare Diseases): http://ord.aspensys.com/asp/diseases/diseases.asp

- Technology Glossary (National Library of Medicine) - Health Care Technology: http://www.nlm.nih.gov/nichsr/ta101/ta10108.htm

Beyond these, MEDLINEplus contains a very patient-friendly encyclopedia covering every aspect of medicine (licensed from A.D.A.M., Inc.). The ADAM Medical Encyclopedia can be accessed at http://www.nlm.nih.gov/medlineplus/encyclopedia.html. ADAM is also available on commercial Web sites such as drkoop.com (http://www.drkoop.com/) and Web MD (http://my.webmd.com/adam/asset/adam_disease_articles/a_to_z/a).

Online Dictionary Directories

The following are additional online directories compiled by the National Library of Medicine, including a number of specialized medical dictionaries:

- Medical Dictionaries: Medical & Biological (World Health Organization): http://www.who.int/hlt/virtuallibrary/English/diction.htm#Medical

- MEL-Michigan Electronic Library List of Online Health and Medical Dictionaries (Michigan Electronic Library): http://mel.lib.mi.us/health/health-dictionaries.html

- Patient Education: Glossaries (DMOZ Open Directory Project): http://dmoz.org/Health/Education/Patient_Education/Glossaries/

- Web of Online Dictionaries (Bucknell University): http://www.yourdictionary.com/diction5.html#medicine

PREMATURE OVARIAN FAILURE DICTIONARY

The definitions below are derived from official public sources, including the National Institutes of Health [NIH] and the European Union [EU].

Abdomen: That portion of the body that lies between the thorax and the pelvis. [NIH]

Aberrant: Wandering or deviating from the usual or normal course. [EU]

Ablation: The removal of an organ by surgery. [NIH]

Abortion: 1. The premature expulsion from the uterus of the products of conception - of the embryo, or of a nonviable fetus. The four classic symptoms, usually present in each type of abortion, are uterine contractions, uterine haemorrhage, softening and dilatation of the cervix, and presentation or expulsion of all or part of the products of conception. 2. Premature stoppage of a natural or a pathological process. [EU]

Acrylonitrile: A highly poisonous compound used widely in the manufacture of plastics, adhesives and synthetic rubber. [NIH]

Adaptability: Ability to develop some form of tolerance to conditions extremely different from those under which a living organism evolved. [NIH]

Adenovirus: A group of viruses that cause respiratory tract and eye infections. Adenoviruses used in gene therapy are altered to carry a specific tumor-fighting gene. [NIH]

Adjuvant: A substance which aids another, such as an auxiliary remedy; in immunology, nonspecific stimulator (e.g., BCG vaccine) of the immune response. [EU]

Adrenal Cortex: The outer layer of the adrenal gland. It secretes mineralocorticoids, androgens, and glucocorticoids. [NIH]

Adrenal Glands: Paired glands situated in the retroperitoneal tissues at the superior pole of each kidney. [NIH]

Adrenal insufficiency: The reduced secretion of adrenal glands. [NIH]

Affinity: 1. Inherent likeness or relationship. 2. A special attraction for a specific element, organ, or structure. 3. Chemical affinity; the force that binds atoms in molecules; the tendency of substances to combine by chemical reaction. 4. The strength of noncovalent chemical binding between two substances as measured by the dissociation constant of the complex. 5. In immunology, a thermodynamic expression of the strength of interaction between a single antigen-binding site and a single antigenic determinant (and thus of the stereochemical compatibility between them), most accurately applied to interactions among simple, uniform antigenic determinants such as haptens. Expressed as the association constant (K litres mole -1), which, owing to the heterogeneity of affinities in a population of antibody molecules of a given specificity, actually represents an average value (mean intrinsic association constant). 6. The reciprocal of the dissociation constant. [EU]

Age of Onset: The age or period of life at which a disease or the initial symptoms or manifestations of a disease appear in an individual. [NIH]

Agonist: In anatomy, a prime mover. In pharmacology, a drug that has affinity for and stimulates physiologic activity at cell receptors normally stimulated by naturally occurring substances. [EU]

Algorithms: A procedure consisting of a sequence of algebraic formulas and/or logical steps to calculate or determine a given task. [NIH]

Alkaline: Having the reactions of an alkali. [EU]

Alleles: Mutually exclusive forms of the same gene, occupying the same locus on homologous chromosomes, and governing the same biochemical and developmental process. [NIH]

Alternative medicine: Practices not generally recognized by the medical community as standard or conventional medical approaches and used instead of standard treatments. Alternative medicine includes the taking of dietary supplements, megadose vitamins, and herbal preparations; the drinking of special teas; and practices such as massage therapy, magnet therapy, spiritual healing, and meditation. [NIH]

Amenorrhea: Absence of menstruation. [NIH]

Amino acid: Any organic compound containing an amino (-NH2 and a carboxyl (- COOH) group. The 20 a-amino acids listed in the accompanying table are the amino acids from which proteins are synthesized by formation of peptide bonds during ribosomal translation of messenger RNA; all except glycine, which is not optically active, have the L configuration. Other amino acids occurring in proteins, such as hydroxyproline in collagen, are formed by posttranslational enzymatic modification of amino acids residues in polypeptide chains. There are also several important amino acids, such as the neurotransmitter y-aminobutyric acid, that have no relation to proteins. Abbreviated AA. [EU]

Amino Acid Sequence: The order of amino acids as they occur in a polypeptide chain. This is referred to as the primary structure of proteins. It is of fundamental importance in determining protein conformation. [NIH]

Amplification: The production of additional copies of a chromosomal DNA sequence, found as either intrachromosomal or extrachromosomal DNA. [NIH]

Anaesthesia: Loss of feeling or sensation. Although the term is used for loss of tactile sensibility, or of any of the other senses, it is applied especially to loss of the sensation of pain, as it is induced to permit performance of surgery or other painful procedures. [EU]

Anal: Having to do with the anus, which is the posterior opening of the large bowel. [NIH]

Analgesic: An agent that alleviates pain without causing loss of consciousness. [EU]

Analog: In chemistry, a substance that is similar, but not identical, to another. [NIH]

Analogous: Resembling or similar in some respects, as in function or appearance, but not in origin or development;. [EU]

Analytes: A component of a test sample the presence of which has to be demonstrated. The term "analyte" includes where appropriate formed from the analyte during the analyses. [NIH]

Anaphylatoxins: The family of peptides C3a, C4a, C5a, and C5a des-arginine produced in the serum during complement activation. They produce smooth muscle contraction, mast cell histamine release, affect platelet aggregation, and act as mediators of the local inflammatory process. The order of anaphylatoxin activity from strongest to weakest is C5a, C3a, C4a, and C5a des-arginine. The latter is the so-called "classical" anaphylatoxin but shows no spasmogenic activity though it contains some chemotactic ability. [NIH]

Androgenic: Producing masculine characteristics. [EU]

Androgens: A class of sex hormones associated with the development and maintenance of the secondary male sex characteristics, sperm induction, and sexual differentiation. In addition to increasing virility and libido, they also increase nitrogen and water retention and stimulate skeletal growth. [NIH]

Androstenedione: A steroid with androgenic properties that is produced in the testis, ovary, and adrenal cortex. It is a precursor to testosterone and other androgenic hormones. [NIH]

Anesthesia: A state characterized by loss of feeling or sensation. This depression of nerve function is usually the result of pharmacologic action and is induced to allow performance of surgery or other painful procedures. [NIH]

Animal model: An animal with a disease either the same as or like a disease in humans. Animal models are used to study the development and progression of diseases and to test new treatments before they are given to humans. Animals with transplanted human cancers or other tissues are called xenograft models. [NIH]

Anions: Negatively charged atoms, radicals or groups of atoms which travel to the anode or positive pole during electrolysis. [NIH]

Anovulation: Suspension or cessation of ovulation in animals and humans. [NIH]

Antiallergic: Counteracting allergy or allergic conditions. [EU]

Antibacterial: A substance that destroys bacteria or suppresses their growth or reproduction. [EU]

Antibiotic: A drug used to treat infections caused by bacteria and other microorganisms. [NIH]

Antibodies: Immunoglobulin molecules having a specific amino acid sequence by virtue of which they interact only with the antigen that induced their synthesis in cells of the lymphoid series (especially plasma cells), or with an antigen closely related to it. [NIH]

Antibody: A type of protein made by certain white blood cells in response to a foreign substance (antigen). Each antibody can bind to only a specific antigen. The purpose of this binding is to help destroy the antigen. Antibodies can work in several ways, depending on the nature of the antigen. Some antibodies destroy antigens directly. Others make it easier for white blood cells to destroy the antigen. [NIH]

Antigen: Any substance which is capable, under appropriate conditions, of inducing a specific immune response and of reacting with the products of that response, that is, with specific antibody or specifically sensitized T-lymphocytes, or both. Antigens may be soluble substances, such as toxins and foreign proteins, or particulate, such as bacteria and tissue cells; however, only the portion of the protein or polysaccharide molecule known as the antigenic determinant (q.v.) combines with antibody or a specific receptor on a lymphocyte. Abbreviated Ag. [EU]

Antigen-Antibody Complex: The complex formed by the binding of antigen and antibody molecules. The deposition of large antigen-antibody complexes leading to tissue damage causes immune complex diseases. [NIH]

Antigen-presenting cell: APC. A cell that shows antigen on its surface to other cells of the immune system. This is an important part of an immune response. [NIH]

Anti-inflammatory: Having to do with reducing inflammation [NIH]

Anti-Inflammatory Agents: Substances that reduce or suppress inflammation. [NIH]

Antineoplastic: Inhibiting or preventing the development of neoplasms, checking the maturation and proliferation of malignant cells. [EU]

Antioxidant: A substance that prevents damage caused by free radicals. Free radicals are highly reactive chemicals that often contain oxygen. They are produced when molecules are split to give products that have unpaired electrons. This process is called oxidation. [NIH]

Anus: The opening of the rectum to the outside of the body. [NIH]

Anxiety: Persistent feeling of dread, apprehension, and impending disaster. [NIH]

Apoptosis: One of the two mechanisms by which cell death occurs (the other being the pathological process of necrosis). Apoptosis is the mechanism responsible for the physiological deletion of cells and appears to be intrinsically programmed. It is characterized by distinctive morphologic changes in the nucleus and cytoplasm, chromatin cleavage at regularly spaced sites, and the endonucleolytic cleavage of genomic DNA (DNA fragmentation) at internucleosomal sites. This mode of cell death serves as a balance to mitosis in regulating the size of animal tissues and in mediating pathologic processes associated with tumor growth. [NIH]

Aquaporins: Membrane proteins which facilitate the passage of water. They are members of the family of membrane channel proteins which includes the lens major intrinsic protein and bacterial glycerol transporters. [NIH]

Arterial: Pertaining to an artery or to the arteries. [EU]

Arteries: The vessels carrying blood away from the heart. [NIH]

Aseptic: Free from infection or septic material; sterile. [EU]

Aspartate: A synthetic amino acid. [NIH]

Aspiration: The act of inhaling. [NIH]

Assay: Determination of the amount of a particular constituent of a mixture, or of the biological or pharmacological potency of a drug. [EU]

Asymptomatic: Having no signs or symptoms of disease. [NIH]

Atresia: Lack of a normal opening from the esophagus, intestines, or anus. [NIH]

Auditory: Pertaining to the sense of hearing. [EU]

Autoantibodies: Antibodies that react with self-antigens (autoantigens) of the organism that produced them. [NIH]

Autoantigens: Endogenous tissue constituents that have the ability to interact with autoantibodies and cause an immune response. [NIH]

Autoimmune disease: A condition in which the body recognizes its own tissues as foreign and directs an immune response against them. [NIH]

Autoimmunity: Process whereby the immune system reacts against the body's own tissues. Autoimmunity may produce or be caused by autoimmune diseases. [NIH]

Bacteria: Unicellular prokaryotic microorganisms which generally possess rigid cell walls, multiply by cell division, and exhibit three principal forms: round or coccal, rodlike or bacillary, and spiral or spirochetal. [NIH]

Basement Membrane: Ubiquitous supportive tissue adjacent to epithelium and around smooth and striated muscle cells. This tissue contains intrinsic macromolecular components such as collagen, laminin, and sulfated proteoglycans. As seen by light microscopy one of its subdivisions is the basal (basement) lamina. [NIH]

Benign: Not cancerous; does not invade nearby tissue or spread to other parts of the body. [NIH]

Bilateral: Affecting both the right and left side of body. [NIH]

Bile: An emulsifying agent produced in the liver and secreted into the duodenum. Its composition includes bile acids and salts, cholesterol, and electrolytes. It aids digestion of fats in the duodenum. [NIH]

Binding Sites: The reactive parts of a macromolecule that directly participate in its specific combination with another molecule. [NIH]

Biochemical: Relating to biochemistry; characterized by, produced by, or involving chemical reactions in living organisms. [EU]

Biological therapy: Treatment to stimulate or restore the ability of the immune system to fight infection and disease. Also used to lessen side effects that may be caused by some cancer treatments. Also known as immunotherapy, biotherapy, or biological response modifier (BRM) therapy. [NIH]

Biological Transport: The movement of materials (including biochemical substances and drugs) across cell membranes and epithelial layers, usually by passive diffusion. [NIH]

Biopsy: Removal and pathologic examination of specimens in the form of small pieces of tissue from the living body. [NIH]

Biosynthesis: The building up of a chemical compound in the physiologic processes of a living organism. [EU]

Biotechnology: Body of knowledge related to the use of organisms, cells or cell-derived constituents for the purpose of developing products which are technically, scientifically and clinically useful. Alteration of biologic function at the molecular level (i.e., genetic engineering) is a central focus; laboratory methods used include transfection and cloning technologies, sequence and structure analysis algorithms, computer databases, and gene and protein structure function analysis and prediction. [NIH]

Bladder: The organ that stores urine. [NIH]

Blastocyst: The mammalian embryo in the post-morula stage in which a fluid-filled cavity, enclosed primarily by trophoblast, contains an inner cell mass which becomes the embryonic disc. [NIH]

Blood Coagulation: The process of the interaction of blood coagulation factors that results in an insoluble fibrin clot. [NIH]

Blood pressure: The pressure of blood against the walls of a blood vessel or heart chamber. Unless there is reference to another location, such as the pulmonary artery or one of the heart chambers, it refers to the pressure in the systemic arteries, as measured, for example, in the forearm. [NIH]

Blood vessel: A tube in the body through which blood circulates. Blood vessels include a network of arteries, arterioles, capillaries, venules, and veins. [NIH]

Blot: To transfer DNA, RNA, or proteins to an immobilizing matrix such as nitrocellulose. [NIH]

Blotting, Western: Identification of proteins or peptides that have been electrophoretically separated by blotting and transferred to strips of nitrocellulose paper. The blots are then detected by radiolabeled antibody probes. [NIH]

Body Fluids: Liquid components of living organisms. [NIH]

Body Mass Index: One of the anthropometric measures of body mass; it has the highest correlation with skinfold thickness or body density. [NIH]

Bone Density: The amount of mineral per square centimeter of bone. This is the definition used in clinical practice. Actual bone density would be expressed in grams per milliliter. It is most frequently measured by photon absorptiometry or x-ray computed tomography. [NIH]

Bone Morphogenetic Proteins: Bone-growth regulatory factors that are members of the transforming growth factor-beta superfamily of proteins. They are synthesized as large precursor molecules which are cleaved by proteolytic enzymes. The active form can consist of a dimer of two identical proteins or a heterodimer of two related bone morphogenetic proteins. [NIH]

Brachytherapy: A collective term for interstitial, intracavity, and surface radiotherapy. It uses small sealed or partly-sealed sources that may be placed on or near the body surface or within a natural body cavity or implanted directly into the tissues. [NIH]

Brain metastases: Cancer that has spread from the original (primary) tumor to the brain. [NIH]

Buccal: Pertaining to or directed toward the cheek. In dental anatomy, used to refer to the buccal surface of a tooth. [EU]

Calcitonin: A peptide hormone that lowers calcium concentration in the blood. In humans, it is released by thyroid cells and acts to decrease the formation and absorptive activity of osteoclasts. Its role in regulating plasma calcium is much greater in children and in certain diseases than in normal adults. [NIH]

Calcium: A basic element found in nearly all organized tissues. It is a member of the alkaline earth family of metals with the atomic symbol Ca, atomic number 20, and atomic weight 40. Calcium is the most abundant mineral in the body and combines with phosphorus to form calcium phosphate in the bones and teeth. It is essential for the normal functioning of nerves and muscles and plays a role in blood coagulation (as factor IV) and in many enzymatic processes. [NIH]

Callus: A callosity or hard, thick skin; the bone-like reparative substance that is formed round the edges and fragments of broken bone. [NIH]

Carbohydrate: An aldehyde or ketone derivative of a polyhydric alcohol, particularly of the pentahydric and hexahydric alcohols. They are so named because the hydrogen and oxygen are usually in the proportion to form water, (CH2O)n. The most important carbohydrates are the starches, sugars, celluloses, and gums. They are classified into mono-, di-, tri-, poly- and heterosaccharides. [EU]

Carcinogenic: Producing carcinoma. [EU]

Cardiac: Having to do with the heart. [NIH]

Case report: A detailed report of the diagnosis, treatment, and follow-up of an individual patient. Case reports also contain some demographic information about the patient (for example, age, gender, ethnic origin). [NIH]

Caspase: Enzyme released by the cell at a crucial stage in apoptosis in order to shred all cellular proteins. [NIH]

Cataracts: In medicine, an opacity of the crystalline lens of the eye obstructing partially or totally its transmission of light. [NIH]

Catheterization: Use or insertion of a tubular device into a duct, blood vessel, hollow organ, or body cavity for injecting or withdrawing fluids for diagnostic or therapeutic purposes. It differs from intubation in that the tube here is used to restore or maintain patency in obstructions. [NIH]

Cell: The individual unit that makes up all of the tissues of the body. All living things are made up of one or more cells. [NIH]

Cell Adhesion: Adherence of cells to surfaces or to other cells. [NIH]

Cell Aggregation: The phenomenon by which dissociated cells intermixed in vitro tend to group themselves with cells of their own type. [NIH]

Cell Death: The termination of the cell's ability to carry out vital functions such as metabolism, growth, reproduction, responsiveness, and adaptability. [NIH]

Cell Differentiation: Progressive restriction of the developmental potential and increasing specialization of function which takes place during the development of the embryo and leads to the formation of specialized cells, tissues, and organs. [NIH]

Cell Division: The fission of a cell. [NIH]

Cell proliferation: An increase in the number of cells as a result of cell growth and cell division. [NIH]

Cell Survival: The span of viability of a cell characterized by the capacity to perform certain functions such as metabolism, growth, reproduction, some form of responsiveness, and adaptability. [NIH]

Central Nervous System: The main information-processing organs of the nervous system, consisting of the brain, spinal cord, and meninges. [NIH]

Centrioles: Self-replicating, short, fibrous, rod-shaped organelles. Each centriole is a short cylinder containing nine pairs of peripheral microtubules, arranged so as to form the wall of the cylinder. [NIH]

Cerebellar: Pertaining to the cerebellum. [EU]

Cerebellar Diseases: Diseases that affect the structure or function of the cerebellum. Cardinal manifestations of cerebellar dysfunction include dysmetria, gait ataxia, and muscle hypotonia. [NIH]

Cerebellum: Part of the metencephalon that lies in the posterior cranial fossa behind the brain stem. It is concerned with the coordination of movement. [NIH]

Cervix: The lower, narrow end of the uterus that forms a canal between the uterus and vagina. [NIH]

Chemotactic Factors: Chemical substances that attract or repel cells or organisms. The concept denotes especially those factors released as a result of tissue injury, invasion, or immunologic activity, that attract leukocytes, macrophages, or other cells to the site of infection or insult. [NIH]

Chemotherapeutic agent: A drug used to treat cancer. [NIH]

Chemotherapy: Treatment with anticancer drugs. [NIH]

Chin: The anatomical frontal portion of the mandible, also known as the mentum, that contains the line of fusion of the two separate halves of the mandible (symphysis menti). This line of fusion divides inferiorly to enclose a triangular area called the mental protuberance. On each side, inferior to the second premolar tooth, is the mental foramen for the passage of blood vessels and a nerve. [NIH]

Cholesterol: The principal sterol of all higher animals, distributed in body tissues, especially the brain and spinal cord, and in animal fats and oils. [NIH]

Choriocarcinoma: A malignant tumor of trophoblastic epithelium characterized by secretion of large amounts of chorionic gonadotropin. It usually originates from chorionic products of conception (i.e., hydatidiform mole, normal pregnancy, or following abortion), but can originate in a teratoma of the testis, mediastinum, or pineal gland. [NIH]

Chromatin: The material of chromosomes. It is a complex of DNA, histones, and nonhistone proteins (chromosomal proteins, non-histone) found within the nucleus of a cell. [NIH]

Chromosomal: Pertaining to chromosomes. [EU]

Chromosome: Part of a cell that contains genetic information. Except for sperm and eggs, all human cells contain 46 chromosomes. [NIH]

Chromosome Abnormalities: Defects in the structure or number of chromosomes resulting in structural aberrations or manifesting as disease. [NIH]

Chromosome Deletion: Actual loss of a portion of the chromosome. [NIH]

Chronic: A disease or condition that persists or progresses over a long period of time. [NIH]

Chronic renal: Slow and progressive loss of kidney function over several years, often resulting in end-stage renal disease. People with end-stage renal disease need dialysis or transplantation to replace the work of the kidneys. [NIH]

Clinical trial: A research study that tests how well new medical treatments or other interventions work in people. Each study is designed to test new methods of screening, prevention, diagnosis, or treatment of a disease. [NIH]

Clomiphene: A stilbene derivative that functions both as a partial estrogen agonist and complete estrogen antagonist depending on the target tissue. It antagonizes the estrogen receptor thereby initiating or augmenting ovulation in anovulatory women. [NIH]

Cloning: The production of a number of genetically identical individuals; in genetic engineering, a process for the efficient replication of a great number of identical DNA molecules. [NIH]

Collagen: A polypeptide substance comprising about one third of the total protein in mammalian organisms. It is the main constituent of skin, connective tissue, and the organic substance of bones and teeth. Different forms of collagen are produced in the body but all consist of three alpha-polypeptide chains arranged in a triple helix. Collagen is differentiated from other fibrous proteins, such as elastin, by the content of proline, hydroxyproline, and hydroxylysine; by the absence of tryptophan; and particularly by the high content of polar groups which are responsible for its swelling properties. [NIH]

Combination chemotherapy: Treatment using more than one anticancer drug. [NIH]

Complement: A term originally used to refer to the heat-labile factor in serum that causes immune cytolysis, the lysis of antibody-coated cells, and now referring to the entire functionally related system comprising at least 20 distinct serum proteins that is the effector not only of immune cytolysis but also of other biologic functions. Complement activation occurs by two different sequences, the classic and alternative pathways. The proteins of the classic pathway are termed 'components of complement' and are designated by the symbols C1 through C9. C1 is a calcium-dependent complex of three distinct proteins C1q, C1r and C1s. The proteins of the alternative pathway (collectively referred to as the properdin system) and complement regulatory proteins are known by semisystematic or trivial names. Fragments resulting from proteolytic cleavage of complement proteins are designated with lower-case letter suffixes, e.g., C3a. Inactivated fragments may be designated with the suffix 'i', e.g. C3bi. Activated components or complexes with biological activity are designated by a bar over the symbol e.g. C1 or C4b,2a. The classic pathway is activated by the binding of C1 to classic pathway activators, primarily antigen-antibody complexes containing IgM, IgG1, IgG3; C1q binds to a single IgM molecule or two adjacent IgG molecules. The alternative pathway can be activated by IgA immune complexes and also by nonimmunologic materials including bacterial endotoxins, microbial polysaccharides, and cell walls. Activation of the classic pathway triggers an enzymatic cascade involving C1, C4, C2 and C3; activation of the alternative pathway triggers a cascade involving C3 and factors B, D and P. Both result in the cleavage of C5 and the formation of the membrane attack complex. Complement activation also results in the formation of many biologically active complement fragments that act as anaphylatoxins, opsonins, or chemotactic factors. [EU]

Complementary and alternative medicine: CAM. Forms of treatment that are used in addition to (complementary) or instead of (alternative) standard treatments. These practices are not considered standard medical approaches. CAM includes dietary supplements, megadose vitamins, herbal preparations, special teas, massage therapy, magnet therapy, spiritual healing, and meditation. [NIH]

Complementary medicine: Practices not generally recognized by the medical community as standard or conventional medical approaches and used to enhance or complement the standard treatments. Complementary medicine includes the taking of dietary supplements, megadose vitamins, and herbal preparations; the drinking of special teas; and practices such as massage therapy, magnet therapy, spiritual healing, and meditation. [NIH]

Computational Biology: A field of biology concerned with the development of techniques for the collection and manipulation of biological data, and the use of such data to make biological discoveries or predictions. This field encompasses all computational methods and theories applicable to molecular biology and areas of computer-based techniques for solving biological problems including manipulation of models and datasets. [NIH]

Conception: The onset of pregnancy, marked by implantation of the blastocyst; the formation of a viable zygote. [EU]

Congenita: Displacement, subluxation, or malposition of the crystalline lens. [NIH]

Congestive heart failure: Weakness of the heart muscle that leads to a buildup of fluid in body tissues. [NIH]

Connective Tissue: Tissue that supports and binds other tissues. It consists of connective tissue cells embedded in a large amount of extracellular matrix. [NIH]

Connective Tissue: Tissue that supports and binds other tissues. It consists of connective tissue cells embedded in a large amount of extracellular matrix. [NIH]

Conscious Sedation: An alternative to general anesthesia in patients for whom general anesthesia is refused or considered inadvisable. It involves the administering of an antianxiety drug (minor tranquilizer) and an analgesic or local anesthetic. This renders the patient free of anxiety and pain while allowing the patient to remain in verbal contact with the physician or dentist. [NIH]

Constitutional: 1. Affecting the whole constitution of the body; not local. 2. Pertaining to the constitution. [EU]

Contraceptive: An agent that diminishes the likelihood of or prevents conception. [EU]

Contraindications: Any factor or sign that it is unwise to pursue a certain kind of action or treatment, e. g. giving a general anesthetic to a person with pneumonia. [NIH]

Controlled study: An experiment or clinical trial that includes a comparison (control) group. [NIH]

Coordination: Muscular or motor regulation or the harmonious cooperation of muscles or groups of muscles, in a complex action or series of actions. [NIH]

Cor: The muscular organ that maintains the circulation of the blood. c. adiposum a heart that has undergone fatty degeneration or that has an accumulation of fat around it; called also fat or fatty, heart. c. arteriosum the left side of the heart, so called because it contains oxygenated (arterial) blood. c. biloculare a congenital anomaly characterized by failure of formation of the atrial and ventricular septums, the heart having only two chambers, a single atrium and a single ventricle, and a common atrioventricular valve. c. bovinum (L. 'ox heart') a greatly enlarged heart due to a hypertrophied left ventricle; called also c. taurinum and bucardia. c. dextrum (L. 'right heart') the right atrium and ventricle. c. hirsutum, c. villosum. c. mobile (obs.) an abnormally movable heart. c. pendulum a heart so movable that it seems to be hanging by the great blood vessels. c. pseudotriloculare biatriatum a congenital cardiac anomaly in which the heart functions as a three-chambered heart because of tricuspid atresia, the right ventricle being extremely small or rudimentary and the right atrium greatly dilated. Blood passes from the right to the left atrium and thence disease due to pulmonary hypertension secondary to disease of the lung, or its blood vessels, with hypertrophy of the right ventricle. [EU]

Cornea: The transparent part of the eye that covers the iris and the pupil and allows light to enter the inside. [NIH]

Coronary: Encircling in the manner of a crown; a term applied to vessels; nerves, ligaments, etc. The term usually denotes the arteries that supply the heart muscle and, by extension, a pathologic involvement of them. [EU]

Coronary Thrombosis: Presence of a thrombus in a coronary artery, often causing a myocardial infarction. [NIH]

Corpus: The body of the uterus. [NIH]

Corpus Luteum: The yellow glandular mass formed in the ovary by an ovarian follicle that has ruptured and discharged its ovum. [NIH]

Cortex: The outer layer of an organ or other body structure, as distinguished from the internal substance. [EU]

Corticosteroid: Any of the steroids elaborated by the adrenal cortex (excluding the sex hormones of adrenal origin) in response to the release of corticotrophin (adrenocorticotropic hormone) by the pituitary gland, to any of the synthetic equivalents of these steroids, or to angiotensin II. They are divided, according to their predominant biological activity, into three major groups: glucocorticoids, chiefly influencing carbohydrate, fat, and protein metabolism; mineralocorticoids, affecting the regulation of electrolyte and water balance; and C19 androgens. Some corticosteroids exhibit both types of activity in varying degrees, and others exert only one type of effect. The corticosteroids are used clinically for hormonal replacement therapy, for suppression of ACTH secretion by the anterior pituitary, as antineoplastic, antiallergic, and anti-inflammatory agents, and to suppress the immune response. Called also adrenocortical hormone and corticoid. [EU]

Crossing-over: The exchange of corresponding segments between chromatids of homologous chromosomes during meiosia, forming a chiasma. [NIH]

Curative: Tending to overcome disease and promote recovery. [EU]

Cutaneous: Having to do with the skin. [NIH]

Cyclic: Pertaining to or occurring in a cycle or cycles; the term is applied to chemical compounds that contain a ring of atoms in the nucleus. [EU]

Cyst: A sac or capsule filled with fluid. [NIH]

Cytokine: Small but highly potent protein that modulates the activity of many cell types, including T and B cells. [NIH]

Cytoplasm: The protoplasm of a cell exclusive of that of the nucleus; it consists of a continuous aqueous solution (cytosol) and the organelles and inclusions suspended in it (phaneroplasm), and is the site of most of the chemical activities of the cell. [EU]

Cytoskeleton: The network of filaments, tubules, and interconnecting filamentous bridges which give shape, structure, and organization to the cytoplasm. [NIH]

Cytotoxic: Cell-killing. [NIH]

Cytotoxic chemotherapy: Anticancer drugs that kill cells, especially cancer cells. [NIH]

Danazol: A synthetic steroid with antigonadotropic and anti-estrogenic activities that acts as an anterior pituitary suppressant by inhibiting the pituitary output of gonadotropins. It possesses some androgenic properties. Danazol has been used in the treatment of endometriosis and some benign breast disorders. [NIH]

Dehydroepiandrosterone: DHEA. A substance that is being studied as a cancer prevention drug. It belongs to the family of drugs called steroids. [NIH]

Deletion: A genetic rearrangement through loss of segments of DNA (chromosomes), bringing sequences, which are normally separated, into close proximity. [NIH]

Dendrites: Extensions of the nerve cell body. They are short and branched and receive stimuli from other neurons. [NIH]

Dendritic: 1. Branched like a tree. 2. Pertaining to or possessing dendrites. [EU]

Dendritic cell: A special type of antigen-presenting cell (APC) that activates T lymphocytes. [NIH]

Density: The logarithm to the base 10 of the opacity of an exposed and processed film. [NIH]

Dermis: A layer of vascular connective tissue underneath the epidermis. The surface of the dermis contains sensitive papillae. Embedded in or beneath the dermis are sweat glands, hair follicles, and sebaceous glands. [NIH]

Detoxification: Treatment designed to free an addict from his drug habit. [EU]

Developmental Biology: The field of biology which deals with the process of the growth and differentiation of an organism. [NIH]

Diagnostic procedure: A method used to identify a disease. [NIH]

Diffusion: The tendency of a gas or solute to pass from a point of higher pressure or concentration to a point of lower pressure or concentration and to distribute itself throughout the available space; a major mechanism of biological transport. [NIH]

Diploid: Having two sets of chromosomes. [NIH]

Direct: 1. Straight; in a straight line. 2. Performed immediately and without the intervention of subsidiary means. [EU]

Disease Susceptibility: A constitution or condition of the body which makes the tissues react in special ways to certain extrinsic stimuli and thus tends to make the individual more than usually susceptible to certain diseases. [NIH]

Disease Vectors: Invertebrates or non-human vertebrates which transmit infective organisms from one host to another. [NIH]

Distal: Remote; farther from any point of reference; opposed to proximal. In dentistry, used to designate a position on the dental arch farther from the median line of the jaw. [EU]

Drive: A state of internal activity of an organism that is a necessary condition before a given stimulus will elicit a class of responses; e.g., a certain level of hunger (drive) must be present before food will elicit an eating response. [NIH]

Duct: A tube through which body fluids pass. [NIH]

Dysgenesis: Defective development. [EU]

Dyspareunia: Painful sexual intercourse. [NIH]

Effector: It is often an enzyme that converts an inactive precursor molecule into an active second messenger. [NIH]

Ejaculation: The release of semen through the penis during orgasm. [NIH]

Elastin: The protein that gives flexibility to tissues. [NIH]

Electrolyte: A substance that dissociates into ions when fused or in solution, and thus becomes capable of conducting electricity; an ionic solute. [EU]

Embryo: The prenatal stage of mammalian development characterized by rapid morphological changes and the differentiation of basic structures. [NIH]

Embryo Transfer: Removal of a mammalian embryo from one environment and replacement in the same or a new environment. The embryo is usually in the pre-nidation phase, i.e., a blastocyst. The process includes embryo or blastocyst transplantation or transfer after in vitro fertilization and transfer of the inner cell mass of the blastocyst. It is not used for transfer of differentiated embryonic tissue, e.g., germ layer cells. [NIH]

Embryogenesis: The process of embryo or embryoid formation, whether by sexual (zygotic) or asexual means. In asexual embryogenesis embryoids arise directly from the explant or on intermediary callus tissue. In some cases they arise from individual cells (somatic cell embryoge). [NIH]

Endemic: Present or usually prevalent in a population or geographical area at all times; said of a disease or agent. Called also endemial. [EU]

Endocrine System: The system of glands that release their secretions (hormones) directly into the circulatory system. In addition to the endocrine glands, included are the chromaffin system and the neurosecretory systems. [NIH]

Endocrinology: A subspecialty of internal medicine concerned with the metabolism, physiology, and disorders of the endocrine system. [NIH]

Endometrial: Having to do with the endometrium (the layer of tissue that lines the uterus). [NIH]

Endometrium: The layer of tissue that lines the uterus. [NIH]

Endotoxins: Toxins closely associated with the living cytoplasm or cell wall of certain microorganisms, which do not readily diffuse into the culture medium, but are released upon lysis of the cells. [NIH]

End-stage renal: Total chronic kidney failure. When the kidneys fail, the body retains fluid and harmful wastes build up. A person with ESRD needs treatment to replace the work of the failed kidneys. [NIH]

Environmental Health: The science of controlling or modifying those conditions, influences, or forces surrounding man which relate to promoting, establishing, and maintaining health. [NIH]

Enzymatic: Phase where enzyme cuts the precursor protein. [NIH]

Enzyme: A protein that speeds up chemical reactions in the body. [NIH]

Enzyme-Linked Immunosorbent Assay: An immunoassay utilizing an antibody labeled with an enzyme marker such as horseradish peroxidase. While either the enzyme or the antibody is bound to an immunosorbent substrate, they both retain their biologic activity; the change in enzyme activity as a result of the enzyme-antibody-antigen reaction is proportional to the concentration of the antigen and can be measured spectrophotometrically or with the naked eye. Many variations of the method have been developed. [NIH]

Epidemic: Occurring suddenly in numbers clearly in excess of normal expectancy; said especially of infectious diseases but applied also to any disease, injury, or other health-related event occurring in such outbreaks. [EU]

Epithelial: Refers to the cells that line the internal and external surfaces of the body. [NIH]

Epithelial Cells: Cells that line the inner and outer surfaces of the body. [NIH]

Epithelium: One or more layers of epithelial cells, supported by the basal lamina, which covers the inner or outer surfaces of the body. [NIH]

Epitopes: Sites on an antigen that interact with specific antibodies. [NIH]

Esophagus: The muscular tube through which food passes from the throat to the stomach. [NIH]

Estradiol: The most potent mammalian estrogenic hormone. It is produced in the ovary, placenta, testis, and possibly the adrenal cortex. [NIH]

Estrogen: One of the two female sex hormones. [NIH]

Estrogen receptor: ER. Protein found on some cancer cells to which estrogen will attach. [NIH]

Estrogen receptor positive: ER+. Breast cancer cells that have a protein (receptor molecule) to which estrogen will attach. Breast cancer cells that are ER+ need the hormone estrogen to grow and will usually respond to hormone (antiestrogen) therapy that blocks these receptor sites. [NIH]

Estrogen Replacement Therapy: The use of hormonal agents with estrogen-like activity in postmenopausal or other estrogen-deficient women to alleviate effects of hormone deficiency, such as vasomotor symptoms, dyspareunia, and progressive development of osteoporosis. This may also include the use of progestational agents in combination therapy. [NIH]

Exogenous: Developed or originating outside the organism, as exogenous disease. [EU]

Expressed Sequence Tags: Sequence tags derived from cDNAs. Expressed sequence tags (ESTs) are partial DNA sequences from clones. [NIH]

External-beam radiation: Radiation therapy that uses a machine to aim high-energy rays at the cancer. Also called external radiation. [NIH]

Extracellular: Outside a cell or cells. [EU]

Extracellular Matrix: A meshwork-like substance found within the extracellular space and in association with the basement membrane of the cell surface. It promotes cellular proliferation and provides a supporting structure to which cells or cell lysates in culture dishes adhere. [NIH]

Extracellular Space: Interstitial space between cells, occupied by fluid as well as amorphous and fibrous substances. [NIH]

Eye Infections: Infection, moderate to severe, caused by bacteria, fungi, or viruses, which occurs either on the external surface of the eye or intraocularly with probable inflammation, visual impairment, or blindness. [NIH]

Fallopian tube: The oviduct, a muscular tube about 10 cm long, lying in the upper border of the broad ligament. [NIH]

Family Planning: Programs or services designed to assist the family in controlling reproduction by either improving or diminishing fertility. [NIH]

Fat: Total lipids including phospholipids. [NIH]

Fetus: The developing offspring from 7 to 8 weeks after conception until birth. [NIH]

Fibronectin: An adhesive glycoprotein. One form circulates in plasma, acting as an opsonin; another is a cell-surface protein which mediates cellular adhesive interactions. [NIH]

Fibrosis: Any pathological condition where fibrous connective tissue invades any organ, usually as a consequence of inflammation or other injury. [NIH]

Flame Retardants: Materials applied to fabrics, bedding, furniture, plastics, etc. to retard their burning; many may leach out and cause allergies or other harm. [NIH]

Follicles: Shafts through which hair grows. [NIH]

Follicular Atresia: The degeneration and resorption of an ovarian follicle before it reaches maturity and ruptures. [NIH]

Follicular Cyst: Cyst due to the occlusion of the duct of a follicle or small gland. [NIH]

Forearm: The part between the elbow and the wrist. [NIH]

FSH: A gonadotropic hormone found in the pituitary tissues of mammals. It regulates the metabolic activity of ovarian granulosa cells and testicular Sertoli cells, induces maturation of Graafian follicles in the ovary, and promotes the development of the germinal cells in the testis. [NIH]

Galactosemia: Buildup of galactose in the blood. Caused by lack of one of the enzymes needed to break down galactose into glucose. [NIH]

Gamete Intrafallopian Transfer: A technique that came into use in the mid-1980's for assisted conception in infertile women with normal fallopian tubes. The protocol consists of hormonal stimulation of the ovaries, followed by laparoscopic follicular aspiration of oocytes, and then the transfer of sperm and oocytes by catheterization into the fallopian tubes. [NIH]

Gas: Air that comes from normal breakdown of food. The gases are passed out of the body through the rectum (flatus) or the mouth (burp). [NIH]

Gastrin: A hormone released after eating. Gastrin causes the stomach to produce more acid. [NIH]

Gelatin: A product formed from skin, white connective tissue, or bone collagen. It is used as a protein food adjuvant, plasma substitute, hemostatic, suspending agent in pharmaceutical preparations, and in the manufacturing of capsules and suppositories. [NIH]

Gene: The functional and physical unit of heredity passed from parent to offspring. Genes are pieces of DNA, and most genes contain the information for making a specific protein. [NIH]

Gene Expression: The phenotypic manifestation of a gene or genes by the processes of gene action. [NIH]

Gene Targeting: The integration of exogenous DNA into the genome of an organism at sites where its expression can be suitably controlled. This integration occurs as a result of homologous recombination. [NIH]

Gene Therapy: The introduction of new genes into cells for the purpose of treating disease by restoring or adding gene expression. Techniques include insertion of retroviral vectors, transfection, homologous recombination, and injection of new genes into the nuclei of single cell embryos. The entire gene therapy process may consist of multiple steps. The new genes may be introduced into proliferating cells in vivo (e.g., bone marrow) or in vitro (e.g., fibroblast cultures) and the modified cells transferred to the site where the gene expression is required. Gene therapy may be particularly useful for treating enzyme deficiency diseases, hemoglobinopathies, and leukemias and may also prove useful in restoring drug sensitivity, particularly for leukemia. [NIH]

Genetic Counseling: Advising families of the risks involved pertaining to birth defects, in order that they may make an informed decision on current or future pregnancies. [NIH]

Genetics: The biological science that deals with the phenomena and mechanisms of heredity. [NIH]

Genital: Pertaining to the genitalia. [EU]

Genotype: The genetic constitution of the individual; the characterization of the genes. [NIH]

Germ Cells: The reproductive cells in multicellular organisms. [NIH]

Gestation: The period of development of the young in viviparous animals, from the time of fertilization of the ovum until birth. [EU]

Gland: An organ that produces and releases one or more substances for use in the body. Some glands produce fluids that affect tissues or organs. Others produce hormones or participate in blood production. [NIH]

Glucocorticoids: A group of corticosteroids that affect carbohydrate metabolism (gluconeogenesis, liver glycogen deposition, elevation of blood sugar), inhibit corticotropin secretion, and possess pronounced anti-inflammatory activity. They also play a role in fat and protein metabolism, maintenance of arterial blood pressure, alteration of the connective tissue response to injury, reduction in the number of circulating lymphocytes, and functioning of the central nervous system. [NIH]

Gluconeogenesis: The process by which glucose is formed from a non-carbohydrate source. [NIH]

Glucose: D-Glucose. A primary source of energy for living organisms. It is naturally occurring and is found in fruits and other parts of plants in its free state. It is used therapeutically in fluid and nutrient replacement. [NIH]

Glycerol: A trihydroxy sugar alcohol that is an intermediate in carbohydrate and lipid metabolism. It is used as a solvent, emollient, pharmaceutical agent, and sweetening agent. [NIH]

Glycine: A non-essential amino acid. It is found primarily in gelatin and silk fibroin and used therapeutically as a nutrient. It is also a fast inhibitory neurotransmitter. [NIH]

Glycogen: A sugar stored in the liver and muscles. It releases glucose into the blood when cells need it for energy. Glycogen is the chief source of stored fuel in the body. [NIH]

Glycoprotein: A protein that has sugar molecules attached to it. [NIH]

Gonad: A sex organ, such as an ovary or a testicle, which produces the gametes in most multicellular animals. [NIH]

Gonadal: Pertaining to a gonad. [EU]

Gonadotropic: Stimulating the gonads; applied to hormones of the anterior pituitary which influence the gonads. [EU]

Gonadotropin: The water-soluble follicle stimulating substance, by some believed to originate in chorionic tissue, obtained from the serum of pregnant mares. It is used to supplement the action of estrogens. [NIH]

Governing Board: The group in which legal authority is vested for the control of health-related institutions and organizations. [NIH]

Granulosa Cells: Cells of the membrana granulosa lining the vesicular ovarian follicle which become luteal cells after ovulation. [NIH]

Gravis: Eruption of watery blisters on the skin among those handling animals and animal products. [NIH]

Growth factors: Substances made by the body that function to regulate cell division and cell survival. Some growth factors are also produced in the laboratory and used in biological therapy. [NIH]

Gynecology: A medical-surgical specialty concerned with the physiology and disorders primarily of the female genital tract, as well as female endocrinology and reproductive physiology. [NIH]

Haematological: Relating to haematology, that is that branch of medical science which treats of the morphology of the blood and blood-forming tissues. [EU]

Haematology: The science of the blood, its nature, functions, and diseases. [NIH]

Haemorrhage: The escape of blood from the vessels; bleeding. Small haemorrhages are classified according to size as petechiae (very small), purpura (up to 1 cm), and ecchymoses (larger). The massive accumulation of blood within a tissue is called a haematoma. [EU]

Heart failure: Loss of pumping ability by the heart, often accompanied by fatigue, breathlessness, and excess fluid accumulation in body tissues. [NIH]

Hemorrhage: Bleeding or escape of blood from a vessel. [NIH]

Hemostasis: The process which spontaneously arrests the flow of blood from vessels carrying blood under pressure. It is accomplished by contraction of the vessels, adhesion and aggregation of formed blood elements, and the process of blood or plasma coagulation. [NIH]

Hepatic: Refers to the liver. [NIH]

Heredity: 1. The genetic transmission of a particular quality or trait from parent to offspring. 2. The genetic constitution of an individual. [EU]

Heterodimer: Zippered pair of nonidentical proteins. [NIH]

Heterozygotes: Having unlike alleles at one or more corresponding loci on homologous chromosomes. [NIH]

Hirsutism: Excess hair in females and children with an adult male pattern of distribution. The concept does not include hypertrichosis, which is localized or generalized excess hair. [NIH]

Histology: The study of tissues and cells under a microscope. [NIH]

Homeobox: Distinctive sequence of DNA bases. [NIH]

Homeostasis: The processes whereby the internal environment of an organism tends to remain balanced and stable. [NIH]

Homodimer: Protein-binding "activation domains" always combine with identical proteins. [NIH]

Homologous: Corresponding in structure, position, origin, etc., as (a) the feathers of a bird and the scales of a fish, (b) antigen and its specific antibody, (c) allelic chromosomes. [EU]

Hormonal: Pertaining to or of the nature of a hormone. [EU]

Hormone: A substance in the body that regulates certain organs. Hormones such as gastrin help in breaking down food. Some hormones come from cells in the stomach and small intestine. [NIH]

Hormone Replacement Therapy: Therapeutic use of hormones to alleviate the effects of hormone deficiency. [NIH]

Hormone therapy: Treatment of cancer by removing, blocking, or adding hormones. Also called endocrine therapy. [NIH]

Horseradish Peroxidase: An enzyme isolated from horseradish which is able to act as an antigen. It is frequently used as a histochemical tracer for light and electron microscopy. Its antigenicity has permitted its use as a combined antigen and marker in experimental immunology. [NIH]

Hybrid: Cross fertilization between two varieties or, more usually, two species of vines, see also crossing. [NIH]

Hydatidiform Mole: A trophoblastic disease characterized by hydrops of the mesenchymal portion of the villus. Its karyotype is paternal and usually homozygotic. The tumor is indistinguishable from chorioadenoma destruens or invasive mole (= hydatidiform mole, invasive) except by karyotype. There is no apparent relation by karyotype to choriocarcinoma. Hydatidiform refers to the presence of the hydropic state of some or all of the villi (Greek hydatis, a drop of water). [NIH]

Hydrogen: The first chemical element in the periodic table. It has the atomic symbol H, atomic number 1, and atomic weight 1. It exists, under normal conditions, as a colorless, odorless, tasteless, diatomic gas. Hydrogen ions are protons. Besides the common H1 isotope, hydrogen exists as the stable isotope deuterium and the unstable, radioactive isotope tritium. [NIH]

Hydrogen Peroxide: A strong oxidizing agent used in aqueous solution as a ripening agent, bleach, and topical anti-infective. It is relatively unstable and solutions deteriorate over time unless stabilized by the addition of acetanilide or similar organic materials. [NIH]

Hydroxylysine: A hydroxylated derivative of the amino acid lysine that is present in certain collagens. [NIH]

Hydroxyproline: A hydroxylated form of the imino acid proline. A deficiency in ascorbic acid can result in impaired hydroxyproline formation. [NIH]

Hyperandrogenism: A state characterized or caused by an excessive secretion of androgens by the adrenal cortex, ovaries, or testes. The clinical significance in males is negligible, so the term is used most commonly with reference to the female. The common manifestations in women are hirsutism and virilism. It is often caused by ovarian disease (particularly the polycystic ovary syndrome) and by adrenal diseases (particularly adrenal gland hyperfunction). [NIH]

Hyperplasia: An increase in the number of cells in a tissue or organ, not due to tumor formation. It differs from hypertrophy, which is an increase in bulk without an increase in the number of cells. [NIH]

Hypersensitivity: Altered reactivity to an antigen, which can result in pathologic reactions upon subsequent exposure to that particular antigen. [NIH]

Hypertrophy: General increase in bulk of a part or organ, not due to tumor formation, nor to an increase in the number of cells. [NIH]

Hypothalamus: Ventral part of the diencephalon extending from the region of the optic chiasm to the caudal border of the mammillary bodies and forming the inferior and lateral walls of the third ventricle. [NIH]

Hypothyroidism: Deficiency of thyroid activity. In adults, it is most common in women and is characterized by decrease in basal metabolic rate, tiredness and lethargy, sensitivity to cold, and menstrual disturbances. If untreated, it progresses to full-blown myxoedema. In infants, severe hypothyroidism leads to cretinism. In juveniles, the manifestations are intermediate, with less severe mental and developmental retardation and only mild symptoms of the adult form. When due to pituitary deficiency of thyrotropin secretion it is called secondary hypothyroidism. [EU]

Idiopathic: Describes a disease of unknown cause. [NIH]

Immune function: Production and action of cells that fight disease or infection. [NIH]

Immune response: The activity of the immune system against foreign substances (antigens). [NIH]

Immune system: The organs, cells, and molecules responsible for the recognition and disposal of foreign ("non-self") material which enters the body. [NIH]

Immunoassay: Immunochemical assay or detection of a substance by serologic or immunologic methods. Usually the substance being studied serves as antigen both in antibody production and in measurement of antibody by the test substance. [NIH]

Immunoblotting: Immunologic methods for isolating and quantitatively measuring immunoreactive substances. When used with immune reagents such as monoclonal antibodies, the process is known generically as western blot analysis (blotting, western). [NIH]

Immunofluorescence: A technique for identifying molecules present on the surfaces of cells or in tissues using a highly fluorescent substance coupled to a specific antibody. [NIH]

Immunoglobulin: A protein that acts as an antibody. [NIH]

Immunologic: The ability of the antibody-forming system to recall a previous experience with an antigen and to respond to a second exposure with the prompt production of large amounts of antibody. [NIH]

Immunology: The study of the body's immune system. [NIH]

Impairment: In the context of health experience, an impairment is any loss or abnormality of psychological, physiological, or anatomical structure or function. [NIH]

Implant radiation: A procedure in which radioactive material sealed in needles, seeds, wires, or catheters is placed directly into or near the tumor. Also called [NIH]

Implantation: The insertion or grafting into the body of biological, living, inert, or radioactive material. [EU]

In situ: In the natural or normal place; confined to the site of origin without invasion of neighbouring tissues. [EU]

In vitro: In the laboratory (outside the body). The opposite of in vivo (in the body). [NIH]

In vivo: In the body. The opposite of in vitro (outside the body or in the laboratory). [NIH]

Incontinence: Inability to control the flow of urine from the bladder (urinary incontinence) or the escape of stool from the rectum (fecal incontinence). [NIH]

Induction: The act or process of inducing or causing to occur, especially the production of a specific morphogenetic effect in the developing embryo through the influence of evocators or organizers, or the production of anaesthesia or unconsciousness by use of appropriate agents. [EU]

Infarction: A pathological process consisting of a sudden insufficient blood supply to an area, which results in necrosis of that area. It is usually caused by a thrombus, an embolus, or a vascular torsion. [NIH]

Infection: 1. Invasion and multiplication of microorganisms in body tissues, which may be clinically unapparent or result in local cellular injury due to competitive metabolism, toxins, intracellular replication, or antigen-antibody response. The infection may remain localized, subclinical, and temporary if the body's defensive mechanisms are effective. A local infection may persist and spread by extension to become an acute, subacute, or chronic clinical infection or disease state. A local infection may also become systemic when the microorganisms gain access to the lymphatic or vascular system. 2. An infectious disease. [EU]

Infertility: The diminished or absent ability to conceive or produce an offspring while sterility is the complete inability to conceive or produce an offspring. [NIH]

Infiltration: The diffusion or accumulation in a tissue or cells of substances not normal to it or in amounts of the normal. Also, the material so accumulated. [EU]

Inflammation: A pathological process characterized by injury or destruction of tissues caused by a variety of cytologic and chemical reactions. It is usually manifested by typical signs of pain, heat, redness, swelling, and loss of function. [NIH]

Inhibin: Glyceroprotein hormone produced in the seminiferous tubules by the Sertoli cells in the male and by the granulosa cells in the female follicles. The hormone inhibits FSH and LH synthesis and secretion by the pituitary cells thereby affecting sexual maturation and fertility. [NIH]

Initiation: Mutation induced by a chemical reactive substance causing cell changes; being a step in a carcinogenic process. [NIH]

Insecticides: Pesticides designed to control insects that are harmful to man. The insects may be directly harmful, as those acting as disease vectors, or indirectly harmful, as destroyers of crops, food products, or textile fabrics. [NIH]

Insertional: A technique in which foreign DNA is cloned into a restriction site which occupies a position within the coding sequence of a gene in the cloning vector molecule. Insertion interrupts the gene's sequence such that its original function is no longer expressed. [NIH]

Insight: The capacity to understand one's own motives, to be aware of one's own psychodynamics, to appreciate the meaning of symbolic behavior. [NIH]

Insomnia: Difficulty in going to sleep or getting enough sleep. [NIH]

Insulin: A protein hormone secreted by beta cells of the pancreas. Insulin plays a major role in the regulation of glucose metabolism, generally promoting the cellular utilization of glucose. It is also an important regulator of protein and lipid metabolism. Insulin is used as a drug to control insulin-dependent diabetes mellitus. [NIH]

Insulin-dependent diabetes mellitus: A disease characterized by high levels of blood glucose resulting from defects in insulin secretion, insulin action, or both. Autoimmune, genetic, and environmental factors are involved in the development of type I diabetes. [NIH]

Integrins: A family of transmembrane glycoproteins consisting of noncovalent heterodimers. They interact with a wide variety of ligands including extracellular matrix glycoproteins, complement, and other cells, while their intracellular domains interact with the cytoskeleton. The integrins consist of at least three identified families: the cytoadhesin receptors, the leukocyte adhesion receptors, and the very-late-antigen receptors. Each family contains a common beta-subunit combined with one or more distinct alpha-subunits. These receptors participate in cell-matrix and cell-cell adhesion in many physiologically important processes, including embryological development, hemostasis, thrombosis, wound healing, immune and nonimmune defense mechanisms, and oncogenic transformation. [NIH]

Intermittent: Occurring at separated intervals; having periods of cessation of activity. [EU]

Internal radiation: A procedure in which radioactive material sealed in needles, seeds, wires, or catheters is placed directly into or near the tumor. Also called brachytherapy, implant radiation, or interstitial radiation therapy. [NIH]

Interstitial: Pertaining to or situated between parts or in the interspaces of a tissue. [EU]

Intestines: The section of the alimentary canal from the stomach to the anus. It includes the large intestine and small intestine. [NIH]

Intracellular: Inside a cell. [NIH]

Intrinsic: Situated entirely within or pertaining exclusively to a part. [EU]

Irradiation: The use of high-energy radiation from x-rays, neutrons, and other sources to kill cancer cells and shrink tumors. Radiation may come from a machine outside the body (external-beam radiation therapy) or from materials called radioisotopes. Radioisotopes produce radiation and can be placed in or near the tumor or in the area near cancer cells. This type of radiation treatment is called internal radiation therapy, implant radiation, interstitial radiation, or brachytherapy. Systemic radiation therapy uses a radioactive substance, such as a radiolabeled monoclonal antibody, that circulates throughout the body. Irradiation is also called radiation therapy, radiotherapy, and x-ray therapy. [NIH]

Kb: A measure of the length of DNA fragments, 1 Kb = 1000 base pairs. The largest DNA fragments are up to 50 kilobases long. [NIH]

Keratoconjunctivitis: Simultaneous inflammation of the cornea and conjunctiva. [NIH]

Keratoconjunctivitis Sicca: Drying and inflammation of the conjunctiva as a result of insufficient lacrimal secretion. When found in association with xerostomia and polyarthritis, it is called Sjogren's syndrome. [NIH]

Labile: 1. Gliding; moving from point to point over the surface; unstable; fluctuating. 2. Chemically unstable. [EU]

Lacrimal: Pertaining to the tears. [EU]

Lactation: The period of the secretion of milk. [EU]

Laminin: Large, noncollagenous glycoprotein with antigenic properties. It is localized in the basement membrane lamina lucida and functions to bind epithelial cells to the basement membrane. Evidence suggests that the protein plays a role in tumor invasion. [NIH]

Latent: Phoria which occurs at one distance or another and which usually has no troublesome effect. [NIH]

Lens: The transparent, double convex (outward curve on both sides) structure suspended between the aqueous and vitreous; helps to focus light on the retina. [NIH]

Lethargy: Abnormal drowsiness or stupor; a condition of indifference. [EU]

Leukocytes: White blood cells. These include granular leukocytes (basophils, eosinophils, and neutrophils) as well as non-granular leukocytes (lymphocytes and monocytes). [NIH]

Libido: The psychic drive or energy associated with sexual instinct in the broad sense (pleasure and love-object seeking). It may also connote the psychic energy associated with instincts in general that motivate behavior. [NIH]

Ligands: A RNA simulation method developed by the MIT. [NIH]

Lipid: Fat. [NIH]

Lipid Peroxidation: Peroxidase catalyzed oxidation of lipids using hydrogen peroxide as an electron acceptor. [NIH]

Liver: A large, glandular organ located in the upper abdomen. The liver cleanses the blood and aids in digestion by secreting bile. [NIH]

Localized: Cancer which has not metastasized yet. [NIH]

Longitudinal study: Also referred to as a "cohort study" or "prospective study"; the analytic method of epidemiologic study in which subsets of a defined population can be identified who are, have been, or in the future may be exposed or not exposed, or exposed in different degrees, to a factor or factors hypothesized to influence the probability of occurrence of a given disease or other outcome. The main feature of this type of study is to observe large numbers of subjects over an extended time, with comparisons of incidence rates in groups that differ in exposure levels. [NIH]

Lucida: An instrument, invented by Wollaton, consisting essentially of a prism or a mirror through which an object can be viewed so as to appear on a plane surface seen in direct view and on which the outline of the object may be traced. [NIH]

Lupus: A form of cutaneous tuberculosis. It is seen predominantly in women and typically involves the nasal, buccal, and conjunctival mucosa. [NIH]

Lymphocyte: A white blood cell. Lymphocytes have a number of roles in the immune system, including the production of antibodies and other substances that fight infection and diseases. [NIH]

Lymphocyte Subsets: A classification of lymphocytes based on structurally or functionally different populations of cells. [NIH]

Lymphocytic: Referring to lymphocytes, a type of white blood cell. [NIH]

Lymphoid: Referring to lymphocytes, a type of white blood cell. Also refers to tissue in which lymphocytes develop. [NIH]

Lymphoma: A general term for various neoplastic diseases of the lymphoid tissue. [NIH]

Lysine: An essential amino acid. It is often added to animal feed. [NIH]

Major Histocompatibility Complex: The genetic region which contains the loci of genes which determine the structure of the serologically defined (SD) and lymphocyte-defined (LD) transplantation antigens, genes which control the structure of the immune response-associated (Ia) antigens, the immune response (Ir) genes which control the ability of an animal to respond immunologically to antigenic stimuli, and genes which determine the structure and/or level of the first four components of complement. [NIH]

Malformation: A morphologic defect resulting from an intrinsically abnormal developmental process. [EU]

Malignancy: A cancerous tumor that can invade and destroy nearby tissue and spread to other parts of the body. [NIH]

Malignant: Cancerous; a growth with a tendency to invade and destroy nearby tissue and spread to other parts of the body. [NIH]

Malignant tumor: A tumor capable of metastasizing. [NIH]

Mammary: Pertaining to the mamma, or breast. [EU]

Manifest: Being the part or aspect of a phenomenon that is directly observable : concretely expressed in behaviour. [EU]

Mediastinum: The area between the lungs. The organs in this area include the heart and its large blood vessels, the trachea, the esophagus, the bronchi, and lymph nodes. [NIH]

MEDLINE: An online database of MEDLARS, the computerized bibliographic Medical Literature Analysis and Retrieval System of the National Library of Medicine. [NIH]

Medroxyprogesterone: (6 alpha)-17-Hydroxy-6-methylpregn-4-ene-3,20-dione. A synthetic progestational hormone used in veterinary practice as an estrus regulator. [NIH]

Medroxyprogesterone Acetate: An injectable contraceptive, generally marketed under the name Depo-Provera. [NIH]

Membrane: A very thin layer of tissue that covers a surface. [NIH]

Menarche: The establishment or beginning of the menstrual function. [EU]

Menopause: Permanent cessation of menstruation. [NIH]

Menstruation: The normal physiologic discharge through the vagina of blood and mucosal tissues from the nonpregnant uterus. [NIH]

Mental: Pertaining to the mind; psychic. 2. (L. mentum chin) pertaining to the chin. [EU]

Mental Health: The state wherein the person is well adjusted. [NIH]

Mental Retardation: Refers to sub-average general intellectual functioning which originated during the developmental period and is associated with impairment in adaptive behavior. [NIH]

Metabolite: Any substance produced by metabolism or by a metabolic process. [EU]

MI: Myocardial infarction. Gross necrosis of the myocardium as a result of interruption of the blood supply to the area; it is almost always caused by atherosclerosis of the coronary arteries, upon which coronary thrombosis is usually superimposed. [NIH]

Microbe: An organism which cannot be observed with the naked eye; e. g. unicellular animals, lower algae, lower fungi, bacteria. [NIH]

Microorganism: An organism that can be seen only through a microscope. Microorganisms include bacteria, protozoa, algae, and fungi. Although viruses are not considered living organisms, they are sometimes classified as microorganisms. [NIH]

Migration: The systematic movement of genes between populations of the same species, geographic race, or variety. [NIH]

Milliliter: A measure of volume for a liquid. A milliliter is approximately 950-times smaller than a quart and 30-times smaller than a fluid ounce. A milliliter of liquid and a cubic centimeter (cc) of liquid are the same. [NIH]

Mineralization: The action of mineralizing; the state of being mineralized. [EU]

Mineralocorticoids: A group of corticosteroids primarily associated with the regulation of water and electrolyte balance. This is accomplished through the effect on ion transport in renal tubules, resulting in retention of sodium and loss of potassium. Mineralocorticoid secretion is itself regulated by plasma volume, serum potassium, and angiotensin II. [NIH]

Mitosis: A method of indirect cell division by means of which the two daughter nuclei normally receive identical complements of the number of chromosomes of the somatic cells of the species. [NIH]

Modeling: A treatment procedure whereby the therapist presents the target behavior which the learner is to imitate and make part of his repertoire. [NIH]

Molecular: Of, pertaining to, or composed of molecules : a very small mass of matter. [EU]

Molecule: A chemical made up of two or more atoms. The atoms in a molecule can be the same (an oxygen molecule has two oxygen atoms) or different (a water molecule has two hydrogen atoms and one oxygen atom). Biological molecules, such as proteins and DNA, can be made up of many thousands of atoms. [NIH]

Monitor: An apparatus which automatically records such physiological signs as respiration, pulse, and blood pressure in an anesthetized patient or one undergoing surgical or other procedures. [NIH]

Monoclonal: An antibody produced by culturing a single type of cell. It therefore consists of a single species of immunoglobulin molecules. [NIH]

Monoclonal antibodies: Laboratory-produced substances that can locate and bind to cancer cells wherever they are in the body. Many monoclonal antibodies are used in cancer detection or therapy; each one recognizes a different protein on certain cancer cells. Monoclonal antibodies can be used alone, or they can be used to deliver drugs, toxins, or radioactive material directly to a tumor. [NIH]

Monocyte: A type of white blood cell. [NIH]

Mononuclear: A cell with one nucleus. [NIH]

Monosomy: The condition in which one chromosome of a pair is missing. In a normally diploid cell it is represented symbolically as 2N-1. [NIH]

Morphological: Relating to the configuration or the structure of live organs. [NIH]

Morphology: The science of the form and structure of organisms (plants, animals, and other forms of life). [NIH]

Mosaicism: The occurrence in an individual of two or more cell populations of different chromosomal constitutions, derived from a single zygote, as opposed to chimerism in which the different cell populations are derived from more than one zygote. [NIH]

Mucosa: A mucous membrane, or tunica mucosa. [EU]

Myasthenia: Muscular debility; any constitutional anomaly of muscle. [EU]

Myocardium: The muscle tissue of the heart composed of striated, involuntary muscle known as cardiac muscle. [NIH]

Necrosis: A pathological process caused by the progressive degradative action of enzymes that is generally associated with severe cellular trauma. It is characterized by mitochondrial swelling, nuclear flocculation, uncontrolled cell lysis, and ultimately cell death. [NIH]

Neoplastic: Pertaining to or like a neoplasm (= any new and abnormal growth); pertaining to neoplasia (= the formation of a neoplasm). [EU]

Nervous System: The entire nerve apparatus composed of the brain, spinal cord, nerves and ganglia. [NIH]

Neuroendocrine: Having to do with the interactions between the nervous system and the endocrine system. Describes certain cells that release hormones into the blood in response to stimulation of the nervous system. [NIH]

Neutrons: Electrically neutral elementary particles found in all atomic nuclei except light hydrogen; the mass is equal to that of the proton and electron combined and they are unstable when isolated from the nucleus, undergoing beta decay. Slow, thermal, epithermal, and fast neutrons refer to the energy levels with which the neutrons are ejected from heavier nuclei during their decay. [NIH]

Nidation: Implantation of the conceptus in the endometrium. [EU]

Nitrogen: An element with the atomic symbol N, atomic number 7, and atomic weight 14. Nitrogen exists as a diatomic gas and makes up about 78% of the earth's atmosphere by volume. It is a constituent of proteins and nucleic acids and found in all living cells. [NIH]

Nuclear: A test of the structure, blood flow, and function of the kidneys. The doctor injects a mildly radioactive solution into an arm vein and uses x-rays to monitor its progress through the kidneys. [NIH]

Nucleus: A body of specialized protoplasm found in nearly all cells and containing the chromosomes. [NIH]

Oestradiol: Growth hormone. [NIH]

Oestrogen: A generic term for oestrus-producing steroid compounds; the female sex hormones. In humans, oestrogen is formed in the ovary, possibly the adrenal cortex, the testis, and the foetoplacental unit; it has various functions in both sexes. It is responsible for the development of the female secondary sex characteristics, and during the menstrual cycle it acts on the female genitalia to produce an environment suitable for the fertilization, implantation, and nutrition of the early embryo. Oestrogen is used in oral contraceptives and as a palliative in cancer of the breast after menopause and cancer of the prostate; other uses include the relief of the discomforts of menopause, inhibition of lactation, and treatment of osteoporosis, threatened abortion, and various functional ovarian disorders. [EU]

Oligomenorrhea: Abnormally infrequent menstruation. [NIH]

Oncogenic: Chemical, viral, radioactive or other agent that causes cancer; carcinogenic. [NIH]

Oocytes: Female germ cells in stages between the prophase of the first maturation division and the completion of the second maturation division. [NIH]

Oogenesis: The formation, development, and maturation of the female germ cell. [NIH]

Opacity: Degree of density (area most dense taken for reading). [NIH]

Osteoclasts: A large multinuclear cell associated with the absorption and removal of bone. An odontoclast, also called cementoclast, is cytomorphologically the same as an osteoclast and is involved in cementum resorption. [NIH]

Osteoporosis: Reduction of bone mass without alteration in the composition of bone, leading to fractures. Primary osteoporosis can be of two major types: postmenopausal osteoporosis and age-related (or senile) osteoporosis. [NIH]

Ovarian Follicle: Spheroidal cell aggregation in the ovary containing an ovum. It consists of an external fibro-vascular coat, an internal coat of nucleated cells, and a transparent, albuminous fluid in which the ovum is suspended. [NIH]

Ovaries: The pair of female reproductive glands in which the ova, or eggs, are formed. The ovaries are located in the pelvis, one on each side of the uterus. [NIH]

Ovary: Either of the paired glands in the female that produce the female germ cells and secrete some of the female sex hormones. [NIH]

Ovulation: The discharge of a secondary oocyte from a ruptured graafian follicle. [NIH]

Ovulation Induction: Techniques for the artifical induction of ovulation. [NIH]

Ovum: A female germ cell extruded from the ovary at ovulation. [NIH]

Oxidation: The act of oxidizing or state of being oxidized. Chemically it consists in the increase of positive charges on an atom or the loss of negative charges. Most biological oxidations are accomplished by the removal of a pair of hydrogen atoms (dehydrogenation) from a molecule. Such oxidations must be accompanied by reduction of an acceptor molecule. Univalent o. indicates loss of one electron; divalent o., the loss of two electrons. [EU]

Oxidative Stress: A disturbance in the prooxidant-antioxidant balance in favor of the former, leading to potential damage. Indicators of oxidative stress include damaged DNA bases, protein oxidation products, and lipid peroxidation products (Sies, Oxidative Stress, 1991, pxv-xvi). [NIH]

Palliative: 1. Affording relief, but not cure. 2. An alleviating medicine. [EU]

Pancreas: A mixed exocrine and endocrine gland situated transversely across the posterior abdominal wall in the epigastric and hypochondriac regions. The endocrine portion is comprised of the Islets of Langerhans, while the exocrine portion is a compound acinar gland that secretes digestive enzymes. [NIH]

Partial remission: The shrinking, but not complete disappearance, of a tumor in response to therapy. Also called partial response. [NIH]

Patch: A piece of material used to cover or protect a wound, an injured part, etc.: a patch over the eye. [NIH]

Pathogenesis: The cellular events and reactions that occur in the development of disease. [NIH]

Pathologic: 1. Indicative of or caused by a morbid condition. 2. Pertaining to pathology (= branch of medicine that treats the essential nature of the disease, especially the structural and functional changes in tissues and organs of the body caused by the disease). [EU]

Pathologic Processes: The abnormal mechanisms and forms involved in the dysfunctions of tissues and organs. [NIH]

Pathophysiology: Altered functions in an individual or an organ due to disease. [NIH]

Patient Education: The teaching or training of patients concerning their own health needs. [NIH]

Pelvis: The lower part of the abdomen, located between the hip bones. [NIH]

Pentoxifylline: A methylxanthine derivative that inhibits phosphodiesterase and affects blood rheology. It improves blood flow by increasing erythrocyte and leukocyte flexibility. It also inhibits platelet aggregation. Pentoxifylline modulates immunologic activity by stimulating cytokine production. [NIH]

Peptide: Any compound consisting of two or more amino acids, the building blocks of proteins. Peptides are combined to make proteins. [NIH]

Peripheral blood: Blood circulating throughout the body. [NIH]

PH: The symbol relating the hydrogen ion (H+) concentration or activity of a solution to that of a given standard solution. Numerically the pH is approximately equal to the negative logarithm of H+ concentration expressed in molarity. pH 7 is neutral; above it alkalinity increases and below it acidity increases. [EU]

Pharmacologic: Pertaining to pharmacology or to the properties and reactions of drugs. [EU]

Phenotype: The outward appearance of the individual. It is the product of interactions between genes and between the genotype and the environment. This includes the killer phenotype, characteristic of yeasts. [NIH]

Phosphodiesterase: Effector enzyme that regulates the levels of a second messenger, the cyclic GMP. [NIH]

Phosphorus: A non-metallic element that is found in the blood, muscles, nevers, bones, and teeth, and is a component of adenosine triphosphate (ATP; the primary energy source for the body's cells.) [NIH]

Phosphorylation: The introduction of a phosphoryl group into a compound through the formation of an ester bond between the compound and a phosphorus moiety. [NIH]

Physiologic: Having to do with the functions of the body. When used in the phrase "physiologic age," it refers to an age assigned by general health, as opposed to calendar age. [NIH]

Physiology: The science that deals with the life processes and functions of organismus, their cells, tissues, and organs. [NIH]

Pineal gland: A tiny organ located in the cerebrum that produces melatonin. Also called pineal body or pineal organ. [NIH]

Pituitary Gland: A small, unpaired gland situated in the sella turcica tissue. It is connected to the hypothalamus by a short stalk. [NIH]

Placenta: A highly vascular fetal organ through which the fetus absorbs oxygen and other nutrients and excretes carbon dioxide and other wastes. It begins to form about the eighth day of gestation when the blastocyst adheres to the decidua. [NIH]

Plants: Multicellular, eukaryotic life forms of the kingdom Plantae. They are characterized by a mainly photosynthetic mode of nutrition; essentially unlimited growth at localized regions of cell divisions (meristems); cellulose within cells providing rigidity; the absence of organs of locomotion; absense of nervous and sensory systems; and an alteration of haploid and diploid generations. [NIH]

Plasma: The clear, yellowish, fluid part of the blood that carries the blood cells. The proteins that form blood clots are in plasma. [NIH]

Plasma cells: A type of white blood cell that produces antibodies. [NIH]

Plasticizers: Materials incorporated mechanically in plastics (usually PVC) to increase flexibility, workability or distensibility; due to the non-chemical inclusion, plasticizers leach out from the plastic and are found in body fluids and the general environment. [NIH]

Platelet Aggregation: The attachment of platelets to one another. This clumping together can be induced by a number of agents (e.g., thrombin, collagen) and is part of the mechanism leading to the formation of a thrombus. [NIH]

Pneumonia: Inflammation of the lungs. [NIH]

Polyarthritis: An inflammation of several joints together. [EU]

Polycystic: An inherited disorder characterized by many grape-like clusters of fluid-filled cysts that make both kidneys larger over time. These cysts take over and destroy working kidney tissue. PKD may cause chronic renal failure and end-stage renal disease. [NIH]

Polycystic Ovary Syndrome: Clinical symptom complex characterized by oligomenorrhea or amenorrhea, anovulation, and regularly associated with bilateral polycystic ovaries. [NIH]

Polylysine: A peptide which is a homopolymer of lysine. [NIH]

Polymorphic: Occurring in several or many forms; appearing in different forms at different stages of development. [EU]

Polymorphism: The occurrence together of two or more distinct forms in the same population. [NIH]

Polypeptide: A peptide which on hydrolysis yields more than two amino acids; called tripeptides, tetrapeptides, etc. according to the number of amino acids contained. [EU]

Polysaccharide: A type of carbohydrate. It contains sugar molecules that are linked together chemically. [NIH]

Postmenopausal: Refers to the time after menopause. Menopause is the time in a woman's life when menstrual periods stop permanently; also called "change of life." [NIH]

Postnatal: Occurring after birth, with reference to the newborn. [EU]

Practice Guidelines: Directions or principles presenting current or future rules of policy for the health care practitioner to assist him in patient care decisions regarding diagnosis, therapy, or related clinical circumstances. The guidelines may be developed by government agencies at any level, institutions, professional societies, governing boards, or by the convening of expert panels. The guidelines form a basis for the evaluation of all aspects of health care and delivery. [NIH]

Precursor: Something that precedes. In biological processes, a substance from which another, usually more active or mature substance is formed. In clinical medicine, a sign or symptom that heralds another. [EU]

Predisposition: A latent susceptibility to disease which may be activated under certain conditions, as by stress. [EU]

Premenopausal: Refers to the time before menopause. Menopause is the time of life when a women's menstrual periods stop permanently; also called "change of life." [NIH]

Prenatal: Existing or occurring before birth, with reference to the fetus. [EU]

Presumptive: A treatment based on an assumed diagnosis, prior to receiving confirmatory laboratory test results. [NIH]

Prevalence: The total number of cases of a given disease in a specified population at a designated time. It is differentiated from incidence, which refers to the number of new cases in the population at a given time. [NIH]

Progesterone: Pregn-4-ene-3,20-dione. The principal progestational hormone of the body, secreted by the corpus luteum, adrenal cortex, and placenta. Its chief function is to prepare the uterus for the reception and development of the fertilized ovum. It acts as an antiovulatory agent when administered on days 5-25 of the menstrual cycle. [NIH]

Progression: Increase in the size of a tumor or spread of cancer in the body. [NIH]

Progressive: Advancing; going forward; going from bad to worse; increasing in scope or severity. [EU]

Proline: A non-essential amino acid that is synthesized from glutamic acid. It is an essential component of collagen and is important for proper functioning of joints and tendons. [NIH]

Promoter: A chemical substance that increases the activity of a carcinogenic process. [NIH]

Prophase: The first phase of cell division, in which the chromosomes become visible, the nucleus starts to lose its identity, the spindle appears, and the centrioles migrate toward opposite poles. [NIH]

Prospective study: An epidemiologic study in which a group of individuals (a cohort), all free of a particular disease and varying in their exposure to a possible risk factor, is followed over a specific amount of time to determine the incidence rates of the disease in the exposed and unexposed groups. [NIH]

Prostate: A gland in males that surrounds the neck of the bladder and the urethra. It secretes a substance that liquifies coagulated semen. It is situated in the pelvic cavity behind the lower part of the pubic symphysis, above the deep layer of the triangular ligament, and rests upon the rectum. [NIH]

Protein S: The vitamin K-dependent cofactor of activated protein C. Together with protein C, it inhibits the action of factors VIIIa and Va. A deficiency in protein S can lead to recurrent venous and arterial thrombosis. [NIH]

Proteins: Polymers of amino acids linked by peptide bonds. The specific sequence of amino acids determines the shape and function of the protein. [NIH]

Proteolytic: 1. Pertaining to, characterized by, or promoting proteolysis. 2. An enzyme that promotes proteolysis (= the splitting of proteins by hydrolysis of the peptide bonds with formation of smaller polypeptides). [EU]

Protocol: The detailed plan for a clinical trial that states the trial's rationale, purpose, drug or vaccine dosages, length of study, routes of administration, who may participate, and other aspects of trial design. [NIH]

Psychic: Pertaining to the psyche or to the mind; mental. [EU]

Puberty: The period during which the secondary sex characteristics begin to develop and the capability of sexual reproduction is attained. [EU]

Public Health: Branch of medicine concerned with the prevention and control of disease and disability, and the promotion of physical and mental health of the population on the international, national, state, or municipal level. [NIH]

Public Policy: A course or method of action selected, usually by a government, from among alternatives to guide and determine present and future decisions. [NIH]

Pulmonary: Relating to the lungs. [NIH]

Purines: A series of heterocyclic compounds that are variously substituted in nature and are known also as purine bases. They include adenine and guanine, constituents of nucleic acids, as well as many alkaloids such as caffeine and theophylline. Uric acid is the metabolic end product of purine metabolism. [NIH]

Pyrimidines: A family of 6-membered heterocyclic compounds occurring in nature in a wide variety of forms. They include several nucleic acid constituents (cytosine, thymine, and uracil) and form the basic structure of the barbiturates. [NIH]

Race: A population within a species which exhibits general similarities within itself, but is both discontinuous and distinct from other populations of that species, though not sufficiently so as to achieve the status of a taxon. [NIH]

Radiation: Emission or propagation of electromagnetic energy (waves/rays), or the waves/rays themselves; a stream of electromagnetic particles (electrons, neutrons, protons, alpha particles) or a mixture of these. The most common source is the sun. [NIH]

Radiation therapy: The use of high-energy radiation from x-rays, gamma rays, neutrons, and other sources to kill cancer cells and shrink tumors. Radiation may come from a machine outside the body (external-beam radiation therapy), or it may come from radioactive material placed in the body in the area near cancer cells (internal radiation therapy, implant radiation, or brachytherapy). Systemic radiation therapy uses a radioactive substance, such as a radiolabeled monoclonal antibody, that circulates throughout the body. Also called radiotherapy. [NIH]

Radioactive: Giving off radiation. [NIH]

Radiolabeled: Any compound that has been joined with a radioactive substance. [NIH]

Radiotherapy: The use of ionizing radiation to treat malignant neoplasms and other benign conditions. The most common forms of ionizing radiation used as therapy are x-rays, gamma rays, and electrons. A special form of radiotherapy, targeted radiotherapy, links a cytotoxic radionuclide to a molecule that targets the tumor. When this molecule is an antibody or other immunologic molecule, the technique is called radioimmunotherapy. [NIH]

Randomized: Describes an experiment or clinical trial in which animal or human subjects are assigned by chance to separate groups that compare different treatments. [NIH]

Receptivity: The condition of the reproductive organs of a female flower that permits effective pollination. [NIH]

Receptor: A molecule inside or on the surface of a cell that binds to a specific substance and causes a specific physiologic effect in the cell. [NIH]

Receptors, Steroid: Proteins found usually in the cytoplasm or nucleus that specifically bind steroid hormones and trigger changes influencing the behavior of cells. The steroid receptor-steroid hormone complex regulates the transcription of specific genes. [NIH]

Recombinant: A cell or an individual with a new combination of genes not found together in either parent; usually applied to linked genes. [EU]

Recombination: The formation of new combinations of genes as a result of segregation in crosses between genetically different parents; also the rearrangement of linked genes due to crossing-over. [NIH]

Rectum: The last 8 to 10 inches of the large intestine. [NIH]

Refer: To send or direct for treatment, aid, information, de decision. [NIH]

Refraction: A test to determine the best eyeglasses or contact lenses to correct a refractive error (myopia, hyperopia, or astigmatism). [NIH]

Regimen: A treatment plan that specifies the dosage, the schedule, and the duration of treatment. [NIH]

Remission: A decrease in or disappearance of signs and symptoms of cancer. In partial remission, some, but not all, signs and symptoms of cancer have disappeared. In complete remission, all signs and symptoms of cancer have disappeared, although there still may be cancer in the body. [NIH]

Reproductive cells: Egg and sperm cells. Each mature reproductive cell carries a single set of 23 chromosomes. [NIH]

Resorption: The loss of substance through physiologic or pathologic means, such as loss of dentin and cementum of a tooth, or of the alveolar process of the mandible or maxilla. [EU]

Rheology: The study of the deformation and flow of matter, usually liquids or fluids, and of the plastic flow of solids. The concept covers consistency, dilatancy, liquefaction, resistance to flow, shearing, thixotrophy, and viscosity. [NIH]

Risk factor: A habit, trait, condition, or genetic alteration that increases a person's chance of developing a disease. [NIH]

Rubber: A high-molecular-weight polymeric elastomer derived from the milk juice (latex) of Hevea brasiliensis and other trees. It is a substance that can be stretched at room temperature to atleast twice its original length and after releasing the stress, retractrapidly, and recover its original dimensions fully. Synthetic rubber is made from many different chemicals, including styrene, acrylonitrile, ethylene, propylene, and isoprene. [NIH]

Salivary: The duct that convey saliva to the mouth. [NIH]

Salivary glands: Glands in the mouth that produce saliva. [NIH]

Saponins: Sapogenin glycosides. A type of glycoside widely distributed in plants. Each consists of a sapogenin as the aglycon moiety, and a sugar. The sapogenin may be a steroid or a triterpene and the sugar may be glucose, galactose, a pentose, or a methylpentose. Sapogenins are poisonous towards the lower forms of life and are powerful hemolytics when injected into the blood stream able to dissolve red blood cells at even extreme dilutions. [NIH]

Screening: Checking for disease when there are no symptoms. [NIH]

Secretion: 1. The process of elaborating a specific product as a result of the activity of a gland; this activity may range from separating a specific substance of the blood to the elaboration of a new chemical substance. 2. Any substance produced by secretion. [EU]

Segregation: The separation in meiotic cell division of homologous chromosome pairs and their contained allelomorphic gene pairs. [NIH]

Selective estrogen receptor modulator: SERM. A drug that acts like estrogen on some tissues, but blocks the effect of estrogen on other tissues. Tamoxifen and raloxifene are SERMs. [NIH]

Sella Turcica: A bony prominence situated on the upper surface of the body of the sphenoid bone. It houses the pituitary gland. [NIH]

Semen: The thick, yellowish-white, viscid fluid secretion of male reproductive organs discharged upon ejaculation. In addition to reproductive organ secretions, it contains spermatozoa and their nutrient plasma. [NIH]

Seminiferous tubule: Tube used to transport sperm made in the testes. [NIH]

Senescence: The bodily and mental state associated with advancing age. [NIH]

Senile: Relating or belonging to old age; characteristic of old age; resulting from infirmity of old age. [NIH]

Serine: A non-essential amino acid occurring in natural form as the L-isomer. It is synthesized from glycine or threonine. It is involved in the biosynthesis of purines, pyrimidines, and other amino acids. [NIH]

Serologic: Analysis of a person's serum, especially specific immune or lytic serums. [NIH]

Serum: The clear liquid part of the blood that remains after blood cells and clotting proteins have been removed. [NIH]

Sex Characteristics: Those characteristics that distinguish one sex from the other. The primary sex characteristics are the ovaries and testes and their related hormones. Secondary sex characteristics are those which are masculine or feminine but not directly related to reproduction. [NIH]

Sicca: Failure of lacrimal secretion, keratoconjunctivitis sicca, failure of secretion of the salivary glands and mucous glands of the upper respiratory tract and polyarthritis. [NIH]

Signs and Symptoms: Clinical manifestations that can be either objective when observed by a physician, or subjective when perceived by the patient. [NIH]

Skeletal: Having to do with the skeleton (boney part of the body). [NIH]

Skeleton: The framework that supports the soft tissues of vertebrate animals and protects many of their internal organs. The skeletons of vertebrates are made of bone and/or cartilage. [NIH]

Skin test: A test for an immune response to a compound by placing it on or under the skin. [NIH]

Skull: The skeleton of the head including the bones of the face and the bones enclosing the brain. [NIH]

Small intestine: The part of the digestive tract that is located between the stomach and the large intestine. [NIH]

Soma: The body as distinct from the mind; all the body tissue except the germ cells; all the axial body. [NIH]

Somatic: 1. Pertaining to or characteristic of the soma or body. 2. Pertaining to the body wall in contrast to the viscera. [EU]

Somatic cells: All the body cells except the reproductive (germ) cells. [NIH]

Specialist: In medicine, one who concentrates on 1 special branch of medical science. [NIH]

Species: A taxonomic category subordinate to a genus (or subgenus) and superior to a subspecies or variety, composed of individuals possessing common characters distinguishing them from other categories of individuals of the same taxonomic level. In taxonomic nomenclature, species are designated by the genus name followed by a Latin or Latinized adjective or noun. [EU]

Specificity: Degree of selectivity shown by an antibody with respect to the number and types of antigens with which the antibody combines, as well as with respect to the rates and the extents of these reactions. [NIH]

Spectrum: A charted band of wavelengths of electromagnetic vibrations obtained by refraction and diffraction. By extension, a measurable range of activity, such as the range of bacteria affected by an antibiotic (antibacterial s.) or the complete range of manifestations of a disease. [EU]

Sperm: The fecundating fluid of the male. [NIH]

Spermatozoa: Mature male germ cells that develop in the seminiferous tubules of the testes. Each consists of a head, a body, and a tail that provides propulsion. The head consists mainly of chromatin. [NIH]

Sporadic: Neither endemic nor epidemic; occurring occasionally in a random or isolated manner. [EU]

Sterility: 1. The inability to produce offspring, i.e., the inability to conceive (female s.) or to induce conception (male s.). 2. The state of being aseptic, or free from microorganisms. [EU]

Steroid: A group name for lipids that contain a hydrogenated cyclopentanoperhydrophenanthrene ring system. Some of the substances included in this group are progesterone, adrenocortical hormones, the gonadal hormones, cardiac aglycones, bile acids, sterols (such as cholesterol), toad poisons, saponins, and some of the carcinogenic hydrocarbons. [EU]

Stimulus: That which can elicit or evoke action (response) in a muscle, nerve, gland or other excitable issue, or cause an augmenting action upon any function or metabolic process. [NIH]

Stomach: An organ of digestion situated in the left upper quadrant of the abdomen between the termination of the esophagus and the beginning of the duodenum. [NIH]

Stool: The waste matter discharged in a bowel movement; feces. [NIH]

Stress: Forcibly exerted influence; pressure. Any condition or situation that causes strain or tension. Stress may be either physical or psychologic, or both. [NIH]

Stroke: Sudden loss of function of part of the brain because of loss of blood flow. Stroke may be caused by a clot (thrombosis) or rupture (hemorrhage) of a blood vessel to the brain. [NIH]

Stroma: The middle, thickest layer of tissue in the cornea. [NIH]

Styrene: A colorless, toxic liquid with a strong aromatic odor. It is used to make rubbers, polymers and copolymers, and polystyrene plastics. [NIH]

Subspecies: A category intermediate in rank between species and variety, based on a smaller number of correlated characters than are used to differentiate species and generally conditioned by geographical and/or ecological occurrence. [NIH]

Substance P: An eleven-amino acid neurotransmitter that appears in both the central and peripheral nervous systems. It is involved in transmission of pain, causes rapid contractions of the gastrointestinal smooth muscle, and modulates inflammatory and immune responses. [NIH]

Substrate: A substance upon which an enzyme acts. [EU]

Superoxide: Derivative of molecular oxygen that can damage cells. [NIH]

Superoxide Dismutase: An oxidoreductase that catalyzes the reaction between superoxide anions and hydrogen to yield molecular oxygen and hydrogen peroxide. The enzyme protects the cell against dangerous levels of superoxide. EC 1.15.1.1. [NIH]

Supplementation: Adding nutrients to the diet. [NIH]

Suppression: A conscious exclusion of disapproved desire contrary with repression, in which the process of exclusion is not conscious. [NIH]

Survival Rate: The proportion of survivors in a group, e.g., of patients, studied and followed over a period, or the proportion of persons in a specified group alive at the beginning of a time interval who survive to the end of the interval. It is often studied using life table methods. [NIH]

Tamoxifen: A first generation selective estrogen receptor modulator (SERM). It acts as an agonist for bone tissue and cholesterol metabolism but is an estrogen antagonist in mammary and uterine. [NIH]

Telomere: A terminal section of a chromosome which has a specialized structure and which is involved in chromosomal replication and stability. Its length is believed to be a few hundred base pairs. [NIH]

Temporal: One of the two irregular bones forming part of the lateral surfaces and base of the skull, and containing the organs of hearing. [NIH]

Teratoma: A type of germ cell tumor that may contain several different types of tissue, such as hair, muscle, and bone. Teratomas occur most often in the ovaries in women, the testicles in men, and the tailbone in children. Not all teratomas are malignant. [NIH]

Testicular: Pertaining to a testis. [EU]

Testis: Either of the paired male reproductive glands that produce the male germ cells and the male hormones. [NIH]

Testosterone: A hormone that promotes the development and maintenance of male sex characteristics. [NIH]

Thorax: A part of the trunk between the neck and the abdomen; the chest. [NIH]

Threonine: An essential amino acid occurring naturally in the L-form, which is the active form. It is found in eggs, milk, gelatin, and other proteins. [NIH]

Thrombosis: The formation or presence of a blood clot inside a blood vessel. [NIH]

Thyroid: A gland located near the windpipe (trachea) that produces thyroid hormone, which helps regulate growth and metabolism. [NIH]

Thyroid Gland: A highly vascular endocrine gland consisting of two lobes, one on either side of the trachea, joined by a narrow isthmus; it produces the thyroid hormones which are concerned in regulating the metabolic rate of the body. [NIH]

Thyroiditis: Inflammation of the thyroid gland. [NIH]

Thyrotropin: A peptide hormone secreted by the anterior pituitary. It promotes the growth of the thyroid gland and stimulates the synthesis of thyroid hormones and the release of thyroxine by the thyroid gland. [NIH]

Tissue: A group or layer of cells that are alike in type and work together to perform a specific function. [NIH]

Tomography: Imaging methods that result in sharp images of objects located on a chosen plane and blurred images located above or below the plane. [NIH]

Toxic: Having to do with poison or something harmful to the body. Toxic substances usually cause unwanted side effects. [NIH]

Toxicity: The quality of being poisonous, especially the degree of virulence of a toxic microbe or of a poison. [EU]

Toxicology: The science concerned with the detection, chemical composition, and pharmacologic action of toxic substances or poisons and the treatment and prevention of toxic manifestations. [NIH]

Toxins: Specific, characterizable, poisonous chemicals, often proteins, with specific biological properties, including immunogenicity, produced by microbes, higher plants, or animals. [NIH]

Trachea: The cartilaginous and membranous tube descending from the larynx and branching into the right and left main bronchi. [NIH]

Transcription Factors: Endogenous substances, usually proteins, which are effective in the initiation, stimulation, or termination of the genetic transcription process. [NIH]

Transdermal: Entering through the dermis, or skin, as in administration of a drug applied to the skin in ointment or patch form. [EU]

Transfection: The uptake of naked or purified DNA into cells, usually eukaryotic. It is analogous to bacterial transformation. [NIH]

Transforming Growth Factor beta: A factor synthesized in a wide variety of tissues. It acts synergistically with TGF-alpha in inducing phenotypic transformation and can also act as a negative autocrine growth factor. TGF-beta has a potential role in embryonal development, cellular differentiation, hormone secretion, and immune function. TGF-beta is found mostly as homodimer forms of separate gene products TGF-beta1, TGF-beta2 or TGF-beta3. Heterodimers composed of TGF-beta1 and 2 (TGF-beta1.2) or of TGF-beta2 and 3 (TGF-beta2.3) have been isolated. The TGF-beta proteins are synthesized as precursor proteins. [NIH]

Translating: Conversion from one language to another language. [NIH]

Translocate: The attachment of a fragment of one chromosome to a non-homologous chromosome. [NIH]

Translocation: The movement of material in solution inside the body of the plant. [NIH]

Transplantation: Transference of a tissue or organ, alive or dead, within an individual, between individuals of the same species, or between individuals of different species. [NIH]

Trees: Woody, usually tall, perennial higher plants (Angiosperms, Gymnosperms, and some Pterophyta) having usually a main stem and numerous branches. [NIH]

Tremor: Cyclical movement of a body part that can represent either a physiologic process or a manifestation of disease. Intention or action tremor, a common manifestation of cerebellar diseases, is aggravated by movement. In contrast, resting tremor is maximal when there is no attempt at voluntary movement, and occurs as a relatively frequent manifestation of Parkinson disease. [NIH]

Trophic: Of or pertaining to nutrition. [EU]

Tryptophan: An essential amino acid that is necessary for normal growth in infants and for nitrogen balance in adults. It is a precursor serotonin and niacin. [NIH]

Tuberculosis: Any of the infectious diseases of man and other animals caused by species of Mycobacterium. [NIH]

Tumor Necrosis Factor: Serum glycoprotein produced by activated macrophages and other mammalian mononuclear leukocytes which has necrotizing activity against tumor cell lines and increases ability to reject tumor transplants. It mimics the action of endotoxin but differs from it. It has a molecular weight of less than 70,000 kDa. [NIH]

Type 2 diabetes: Usually characterized by a gradual onset with minimal or no symptoms of metabolic disturbance and no requirement for exogenous insulin. The peak age of onset is 50 to 60 years. Obesity and possibly a genetic factor are usually present. [NIH]

Urinary: Having to do with urine or the organs of the body that produce and get rid of urine. [NIH]

Urine: Fluid containing water and waste products. Urine is made by the kidneys, stored in the bladder, and leaves the body through the urethra. [NIH]

Uterine Contraction: Contraction of the uterine muscle. [NIH]

Uterus: The small, hollow, pear-shaped organ in a woman's pelvis. This is the organ in which a fetus develops. Also called the womb. [NIH]

Vagina: The muscular canal extending from the uterus to the exterior of the body. Also called the birth canal. [NIH]

Vaginal: Of or having to do with the vagina, the birth canal. [NIH]

Vascular: Pertaining to blood vessels or indicative of a copious blood supply. [EU]

Vasomotor: 1. Affecting the calibre of a vessel, especially of a blood vessel. 2. Any element or agent that effects the calibre of a blood vessel. [EU]

Vector: Plasmid or other self-replicating DNA molecule that transfers DNA between cells in nature or in recombinant DNA technology. [NIH]

Vein: Vessel-carrying blood from various parts of the body to the heart. [NIH]

Vesicular: 1. Composed of or relating to small, saclike bodies. 2. Pertaining to or made up of vesicles on the skin. [EU]

Veterinary Medicine: The medical science concerned with the prevention, diagnosis, and treatment of diseases in animals. [NIH]

Virilism: Development of masculine traits in the female. [NIH]

Virulence: The degree of pathogenicity within a group or species of microorganisms or viruses as indicated by case fatality rates and/or the ability of the organism to invade the tissues of the host. [NIH]

Viruses: Minute infectious agents whose genomes are composed of DNA or RNA, but not both. They are characterized by a lack of independent metabolism and the inability to replicate outside living host cells. [NIH]

Viscera: Any of the large interior organs in any one of the three great cavities of the body, especially in the abdomen. [NIH]

Vitro: Descriptive of an event or enzyme reaction under experimental investigation occurring outside a living organism. Parts of an organism or microorganism are used together with artificial substrates and/or conditions. [NIH]

Vivo: Outside of or removed from the body of a living organism. [NIH]

White blood cell: A type of cell in the immune system that helps the body fight infection and disease. White blood cells include lymphocytes, granulocytes, macrophages, and others. [NIH]

Windpipe: A rigid tube, 10 cm long, extending from the cricoid cartilage to the upper border of the fifth thoracic vertebra. [NIH]

Wound Healing: Restoration of integrity to traumatized tissue. [NIH]

Xenograft: The cells of one species transplanted to another species. [NIH]

X-ray: High-energy radiation used in low doses to diagnose diseases and in high doses to treat cancer. [NIH]

X-ray therapy: The use of high-energy radiation from x-rays to kill cancer cells and shrink tumors. Radiation may come from a machine outside the body (external-beam radiation therapy) or from materials called radioisotopes. Radioisotopes produce radiation and can be placed in or near the tumor or in the area near cancer cells. This type of radiation treatment is called internal radiation therapy, implant radiation, interstitial radiation, or brachytherapy. Systemic radiation therapy uses a radioactive substance, such as a radiolabeled monoclonal antibody, that circulates throughout the body. X-ray therapy is also called radiation therapy, radiotherapy, and irradiation. [NIH]

Yeasts: A general term for single-celled rounded fungi that reproduce by budding. Brewers' and bakers' yeasts are Saccharomyces cerevisiae; therapeutic dried yeast is dried yeast. [NIH]

Zona Pellucida: The transport non-cellular envelope surrounding the mammalian ovum. [NIH]

Zygote: The fertilized ovum. [NIH]

INDEX

A

Abdomen, 64, 95, 114, 118, 124, 125, 128
Aberrant, 69, 95
Ablation, 8, 43, 95
Abortion, 60, 95, 101, 117
Acrylonitrile, 95, 123
Adaptability, 95, 100, 101
Adenovirus, 10, 95
Adjuvant, 11, 95, 108
Adrenal Cortex, 95, 97, 104, 106, 111, 117, 120
Adrenal Glands, 95
Adrenal insufficiency, 20, 95
Affinity, 95
Age of Onset, 95, 127
Agonist, 63, 95, 102, 125
Algorithms, 95, 99
Alkaline, 96, 100
Alleles, 5, 96, 110
Alternative medicine, 96
Amenorrhea, 33, 36, 64, 68, 96, 120
Amino acid, 96, 97, 98, 109, 111, 115, 118, 120, 121, 123, 125, 127
Amino Acid Sequence, 96, 97
Amplification, 10, 96
Anaesthesia, 96, 112
Anal, 96, 114
Analgesic, 96, 103
Analog, 17, 96
Analogous, 96, 126
Analytes, 82, 96
Anaphylatoxins, 96, 102
Androgenic, 15, 96, 97, 104
Androgens, 56, 95, 96, 104, 111
Androstenedione, 53, 56, 97
Anesthesia, 97, 103
Animal model, 14, 70, 97
Anions, 97, 125
Anovulation, 97, 120
Antiallergic, 97, 104
Antibacterial, 97, 124
Antibiotic, 97, 124
Antibodies, 12, 19, 20, 21, 24, 25, 33, 39, 51, 97, 98, 106, 114, 116, 119
Antibody, 21, 95, 97, 99, 102, 106, 110, 111, 112, 113, 116, 122, 124, 128
Antigen, 12, 19, 32, 39, 68, 95, 97, 102, 105, 106, 110, 111, 112, 113

Antigen-Antibody Complex, 97, 102
Antigen-presenting cell, 97, 105
Anti-inflammatory, 97, 104, 109
Anti-Inflammatory Agents, 97, 104
Antineoplastic, 97, 104
Antioxidant, 97, 118
Anus, 96, 97, 98, 113
Anxiety, 97, 103
Apoptosis, 7, 13, 16, 98, 100
Aquaporins, 16, 98
Arterial, 98, 103, 109, 121
Arteries, 98, 99, 104, 115
Aseptic, 98, 124
Aspartate, 32, 98
Aspiration, 98, 108
Assay, 25, 98, 111
Asymptomatic, 20, 98
Atresia, 14, 16, 98, 103
Auditory, 25, 98
Autoantibodies, 12, 17, 21, 22, 34, 44, 55, 68, 69, 98
Autoantigens, 12, 98
Autoimmune disease, 12, 17, 35, 50, 98
Autoimmunity, 12, 22, 32, 33, 35, 39, 44, 48, 49, 50, 51, 55, 68, 98

B

Bacteria, 97, 98, 107, 115, 124
Basement Membrane, 98, 107, 114
Benign, 98, 104, 122
Bilateral, 54, 98, 120
Bile, 98, 114, 124
Binding Sites, 15, 98
Biochemical, 7, 33, 96, 98, 99
Biological therapy, 99, 109
Biological Transport, 99, 105
Biopsy, 37, 99
Biosynthesis, 99, 123
Biotechnology, 16, 77, 99
Bladder, 99, 112, 121, 127
Blastocyst, 99, 103, 105, 119
Blood Coagulation, 99, 100
Blood pressure, 99, 109, 116
Blood vessel, 99, 100, 101, 103, 115, 125, 127
Blot, 99, 111
Blotting, Western, 99, 111
Body Fluids, 99, 105, 119
Body Mass Index, 11, 99

Bone Density, 7, 99
Bone Morphogenetic Proteins, 8, 99
Brachytherapy, 99, 113, 122, 128
Brain metastases, 63, 100
Buccal, 100, 114

C

Calcitonin, 11, 100
Calcium, 11, 100, 102
Callus, 100, 106
Carbohydrate, 100, 104, 108, 109, 120
Carcinogenic, 100, 112, 117, 120, 124
Cardiac, 100, 103, 116, 124
Case report, 23, 39, 40, 41, 45, 58, 59, 100
Caspase, 10, 100
Cataracts, 16, 100
Catheterization, 100, 108
Cell Adhesion, 100, 113
Cell Aggregation, 100, 118
Cell Death, 7, 16, 98, 100, 117
Cell Differentiation, 10, 100
Cell Division, 98, 101, 109, 116, 119, 120, 123
Cell proliferation, 14, 101
Cell Survival, 10, 101, 109
Central Nervous System, 101, 109
Centrioles, 101, 121
Cerebellar, 5, 101, 127
Cerebellar Diseases, 101, 127
Cerebellum, 101
Cervix, 95, 101
Chemotactic Factors, 101, 102
Chemotherapeutic agent, 6, 7, 101
Chemotherapy, 11, 24, 51, 62, 63, 69, 101
Chin, 64, 101, 115
Cholesterol, 98, 101, 124, 125
Choriocarcinoma, 63, 101, 110
Chromatin, 98, 101, 124
Chromosomal, 69, 96, 101, 116, 125
Chromosome, 9, 18, 27, 28, 29, 39, 45, 59, 60, 101, 116, 123, 125, 126
Chromosome Abnormalities, 60, 101
Chromosome Deletion, 18, 101
Chronic, 6, 101, 102, 106, 112, 120
Chronic renal, 102, 120
Clinical trial, 3, 77, 102, 103, 121, 122
Clomiphene, 40, 102
Cloning, 99, 102, 113
Collagen, 14, 96, 98, 102, 108, 119, 120
Combination chemotherapy, 63, 102
Complement, 52, 96, 102, 113, 115
Complementary and alternative medicine, 61, 65, 102

Complementary medicine, 61, 102
Computational Biology, 77, 103
Conception, 51, 95, 101, 103, 107, 108, 124
Congenita, 29, 103
Congestive heart failure, 16, 103
Connective Tissue, 102, 103, 105, 107, 108, 109
Conscious Sedation, 37, 103
Constitutional, 103, 116
Contraceptive, 103, 115
Contraindications, ii, 103
Controlled study, 18, 103
Coordination, 10, 101, 103
Cor, 103, 108
Cornea, 103, 113, 125
Coronary, 104, 115
Coronary Thrombosis, 104, 115
Corpus, 104, 120
Corpus Luteum, 104, 120
Cortex, 104
Corticosteroid, 41, 104
Crossing-over, 104, 122
Curative, 63, 104
Cutaneous, 104, 114
Cyclic, 20, 25, 27, 104, 119
Cyst, 16, 104, 107
Cytokine, 104, 118
Cytoplasm, 98, 104, 106, 122
Cytoskeleton, 104, 113
Cytotoxic, 62, 104, 122
Cytotoxic chemotherapy, 62, 104

D

Danazol, 18, 104
Dehydroepiandrosterone, 53, 104
Deletion, 4, 25, 28, 39, 98, 104
Dendrites, 105
Dendritic, 19, 27, 105
Dendritic cell, 19, 27, 105
Density, 7, 11, 27, 99, 105, 117
Dermis, 105, 126
Detoxification, 7, 105
Developmental Biology, 15, 105
Diagnostic procedure, 67, 105
Diffusion, 16, 99, 105, 112
Diploid, 105, 116, 119
Direct, iii, 10, 105, 114, 122
Disease Susceptibility, 12, 105
Disease Vectors, 105, 112
Distal, 9, 105
Drive, ii, vi, 16, 83, 105, 114
Duct, 100, 105, 107, 123
Dysgenesis, 32, 44, 105

Dyspareunia, 68, 105, 107
E
Effector, 102, 105, 119
Ejaculation, 105, 123
Elastin, 102, 105
Electrolyte, 104, 105, 116
Embryo, 41, 42, 53, 55, 95, 99, 100, 105, 106, 112, 117
Embryo Transfer, 41, 42, 53, 55, 105
Embryogenesis, 15, 106
Endemic, 106, 124
Endocrine System, 106, 117
Endometrial, 28, 43, 57, 106
Endometrium, 28, 106, 117
Endotoxins, 102, 106
End-stage renal, 102, 106, 120
Environmental Health, 76, 78, 106
Enzymatic, 96, 100, 102, 106
Enzyme, 33, 100, 105, 106, 108, 110, 119, 121, 125, 128
Enzyme-Linked Immunosorbent Assay, 33, 106
Epidemic, 106, 124
Epithelial, 56, 99, 106, 114
Epithelial Cells, 56, 106, 114
Epithelium, 18, 98, 101, 106
Epitopes, 17, 106
Esophagus, 98, 106, 115, 124
Estradiol, 10, 15, 24, 41, 52, 59, 61, 106
Estrogen, 7, 11, 15, 42, 52, 58, 71, 82, 102, 106, 107, 123, 125
Estrogen receptor, 11, 15, 102, 107
Estrogen receptor positive, 11, 107
Estrogen Replacement Therapy, 7, 42, 107
Exogenous, 107, 108, 127
Expressed Sequence Tags, 15, 107
External-beam radiation, 107, 113, 121, 128
Extracellular, 13, 103, 107, 113
Extracellular Matrix, 13, 103, 107, 113
Extracellular Space, 107
Eye Infections, 95, 107
F
Fallopian tube, 107, 108
Family Planning, 77, 107
Fat, 103, 104, 107, 109, 114
Fetus, 14, 95, 107, 119, 120, 127
Fibronectin, 14, 107
Fibrosis, 16, 107
Flame Retardants, 6, 107
Follicles, 6, 9, 13, 14, 15, 26, 105, 107, 108, 112

Follicular Atresia, 6, 14, 107
Follicular Cyst, 6, 107
Forearm, 11, 99, 107
FSH, 9, 82, 107, 112
G
Galactosemia, 39, 53, 108
Gamete Intrafallopian Transfer, 38, 39, 41, 108
Gas, 105, 108, 110, 117
Gastrin, 108, 110
Gelatin, 108, 109, 125
Gene, 4, 5, 8, 15, 18, 19, 21, 29, 30, 31, 35, 38, 40, 44, 57, 68, 95, 96, 99, 108, 113, 123, 126
Gene Expression, 8, 21, 108
Gene Targeting, 15, 108
Gene Therapy, 95, 108
Genetic Counseling, 9, 108
Genetics, 3, 4, 5, 15, 18, 21, 23, 29, 30, 32, 34, 37, 38, 40, 42, 43, 45, 46, 52, 55, 58, 68, 108
Genital, 70, 108, 109
Genotype, 108, 119
Germ Cells, 13, 69, 108, 117, 118, 124, 125
Gestation, 58, 108, 119
Gland, 4, 95, 107, 108, 111, 118, 119, 121, 123, 124, 125, 126
Glucocorticoids, 32, 95, 104, 108
Gluconeogenesis, 108, 109
Glucose, 108, 109, 113, 123
Glycerol, 98, 109
Glycine, 96, 109, 123
Glycogen, 108, 109
Glycoprotein, 107, 109, 114, 127
Gonad, 109
Gonadal, 7, 13, 19, 62, 109, 124
Gonadotropic, 107, 109
Gonadotropin, 4, 9, 17, 20, 26, 31, 36, 40, 42, 49, 57, 59, 101, 109
Governing Board, 109, 120
Granulosa Cells, 8, 9, 10, 13, 16, 64, 107, 109, 112
Gravis, 23, 38, 53, 109
Growth factors, 15, 109
Gynecology, 9, 13, 17, 23, 24, 25, 26, 34, 36, 40, 41, 42, 43, 44, 46, 48, 49, 50, 53, 54, 58, 59, 109
H
Haematological, 62, 109
Haematology, 109
Haemorrhage, 95, 109
Heart failure, 109

Hemorrhage, 109, 125
Hemostasis, 110, 113
Hepatic, 24, 110
Heredity, 108, 110
Heterodimer, 99, 110
Heterozygotes, 28, 110
Hirsutism, 110, 111
Histology, 6, 15, 110
Homeobox, 15, 110
Homeostasis, 15, 110
Homodimer, 110, 126
Homologous, 15, 32, 96, 104, 108, 110, 123, 126
Hormonal, 9, 24, 26, 59, 104, 107, 108, 110
Hormone Replacement Therapy, 11, 18, 27, 28, 55, 57, 58, 71, 82, 110
Hormone therapy, 34, 110
Horseradish Peroxidase, 106, 110
Hybrid, 62, 110
Hydatidiform Mole, 101, 110
Hydrogen, 100, 110, 111, 114, 116, 117, 118, 119, 125
Hydrogen Peroxide, 111, 114, 125
Hydroxylysine, 102, 111
Hydroxyproline, 96, 102, 111
Hyperandrogenism, 14, 111
Hyperplasia, 6, 111
Hypersensitivity, 20, 111
Hypertrophy, 103, 111
Hypothalamus, 111, 119
Hypothyroidism, 43, 111

I
Idiopathic, 9, 17, 21, 24, 28, 29, 33, 34, 35, 46, 52, 68, 69, 111
Immune function, 111, 126
Immune response, 95, 97, 98, 104, 111, 115, 124, 125
Immune system, 97, 98, 99, 111, 112, 114, 128
Immunoassay, 12, 39, 106, 111
Immunoblotting, 33, 111
Immunofluorescence, 14, 25, 33, 111
Immunoglobulin, 57, 97, 111, 116
Immunologic, 34, 101, 111, 118, 122
Immunology, 20, 24, 27, 33, 34, 35, 62, 95, 110, 112
Impairment, 107, 112, 115
Implant radiation, 112, 113, 122, 128
Implantation, 103, 112, 117
In situ, 11, 112
In vitro, 10, 13, 41, 55, 58, 64, 100, 105, 108, 112

In vivo, 8, 14, 108, 112
Incontinence, 68, 112
Induction, 39, 40, 57, 62, 96, 112, 118
Infarction, 104, 112, 115
Infection, 98, 99, 101, 107, 111, 112, 114, 128
Infertility, 6, 8, 12, 13, 26, 31, 32, 68, 69, 82, 112
Infiltration, 69, 112
Inflammation, 97, 107, 112, 113, 119, 126
Inhibin, 30, 35, 51, 62, 68, 112
Initiation, 112, 126
Insecticides, 6, 112
Insertional, 70, 113
Insight, 5, 6, 7, 9, 10, 13, 15, 113
Insomnia, 68, 113
Insulin, 32, 113, 127
Insulin-dependent diabetes mellitus, 113
Integrins, 14, 113
Intermittent, 68, 113
Internal radiation, 113, 122, 128
Interstitial, 28, 99, 107, 113, 128
Intestines, 98, 113
Intracellular, 9, 16, 112, 113
Intrinsic, 95, 98, 113
Irradiation, 69, 113, 128

K
Kb, 76, 113
Keratoconjunctivitis, 113, 123
Keratoconjunctivitis Sicca, 113, 123

L
Labile, 102, 114
Lacrimal, 113, 114, 123
Lactation, 114, 117
Laminin, 14, 98, 114
Latent, 114, 120
Lens, 98, 100, 103, 114
Lethargy, 111, 114
Leukocytes, 101, 114, 127
Libido, 96, 114
Ligands, 8, 113, 114
Lipid, 16, 109, 113, 114, 118
Lipid Peroxidation, 114, 118
Liver, 98, 108, 109, 110, 114
Localized, 110, 112, 114, 119
Longitudinal study, 7, 114
Lucida, 114
Lupus, 54, 114
Lymphocyte, 20, 27, 34, 35, 36, 97, 114, 115
Lymphocyte Subsets, 20, 27, 34, 114
Lymphocytic, 69, 114
Lymphoid, 97, 114

Lymphoma, 62, 63, 114
Lysine, 111, 115, 120
M
Major Histocompatibility Complex, 35, 115
Malformation, 18, 115
Malignancy, 62, 115
Malignant, 97, 101, 115, 122, 125
Malignant tumor, 101, 115
Mammary, 115, 125
Manifest, 69, 115
Mediastinum, 101, 115
MEDLINE, 77, 115
Medroxyprogesterone, 20, 115
Medroxyprogesterone Acetate, 20, 115
Membrane, 98, 102, 114, 115, 116
Menarche, 68, 115
Menopause, 6, 11, 12, 13, 15, 46, 50, 61, 63, 65, 68, 69, 70, 71, 82, 83, 115, 117, 120
Menstruation, 96, 115, 117
Mental, iv, 3, 4, 5, 76, 78, 101, 111, 115, 121, 123
Mental Health, iv, 3, 76, 78, 115, 121
Mental Retardation, 4, 5, 115
Metabolite, 6, 115
MI, 11, 29, 34, 42, 55, 57, 93, 115
Microbe, 115, 126
Microorganism, 115, 128
Migration, 69, 116
Milliliter, 99, 116
Mineralization, 62, 116
Mineralocorticoids, 95, 104, 116
Mitosis, 98, 116
Modeling, 7, 116
Molecule, 97, 98, 102, 105, 107, 113, 116, 118, 122, 127
Monitor, 116, 117
Monoclonal, 111, 113, 116, 122, 128
Monoclonal antibodies, 111, 116
Monocyte, 19, 116
Mononuclear, 116, 127
Monosomy, 9, 116
Morphological, 7, 50, 105, 116
Morphology, 6, 14, 109, 116
Mosaicism, 17, 60, 116
Mucosa, 114, 116
Myasthenia, 23, 38, 53, 116
Myocardium, 115, 116
N
Necrosis, 98, 112, 115, 116
Neoplastic, 114, 117
Nervous System, 101, 117, 125

Neuroendocrine, 14, 117
Neutrons, 113, 117, 121
Nidation, 105, 117
Nitrogen, 96, 117, 127
Nuclear, 21, 117
Nucleus, 8, 98, 101, 104, 116, 117, 121, 122
O
Oestradiol, 68, 117
Oestrogen, 36, 117
Oligomenorrhea, 117, 120
Oncogenic, 113, 117
Oocytes, 6, 13, 15, 16, 26, 41, 108, 117
Oogenesis, 15, 18, 117
Opacity, 100, 105, 117
Osteoclasts, 100, 117
Osteoporosis, 7, 11, 107, 117
Ovarian Follicle, 14, 104, 107, 109, 118
Ovaries, 6, 9, 15, 24, 51, 56, 69, 83, 108, 111, 118, 120, 123, 125
Ovary, 6, 8, 9, 12, 13, 15, 36, 38, 52, 69, 97, 104, 106, 108, 109, 117, 118
Ovulation, 10, 17, 39, 40, 51, 54, 55, 57, 69, 97, 102, 109, 118
Ovulation Induction, 17, 51, 54, 118
Ovum, 54, 104, 108, 118, 120, 128
Oxidation, 97, 114, 118
Oxidative Stress, 7, 118
P
Palliative, 117, 118
Pancreas, 113, 118
Partial remission, 118, 122
Patch, 118, 126
Pathogenesis, 12, 118
Pathologic, 15, 98, 99, 104, 111, 118, 122
Pathologic Processes, 15, 98, 118
Pathophysiology, 6, 9, 118
Patient Education, 83, 88, 90, 93, 118
Pelvis, 95, 118, 127
Pentoxifylline, 55, 118
Peptide, 96, 100, 118, 120, 121, 126
Peripheral blood, 20, 34, 119
PH, 99, 119
Pharmacologic, 97, 119, 126
Phenotype, 4, 5, 6, 9, 119
Phosphodiesterase, 118, 119
Phosphorus, 100, 119
Phosphorylation, 8, 10, 14, 119
Physiologic, 95, 99, 115, 119, 122, 127
Physiology, 6, 8, 13, 106, 109, 119
Pineal gland, 101, 119
Pituitary Gland, 4, 104, 119, 123
Placenta, 106, 119, 120

Plants, 109, 116, 119, 123, 126
Plasma, 27, 97, 100, 107, 108, 110, 116, 119, 123
Plasma cells, 97, 119
Plasticizers, 6, 119
Platelet Aggregation, 96, 118, 119
Pneumonia, 103, 119
Polyarthritis, 113, 119, 123
Polycystic, 8, 10, 19, 24, 29, 37, 38, 111, 119, 120
Polycystic Ovary Syndrome, 8, 19, 29, 37, 38, 111, 120
Polylysine, 14, 120
Polymorphic, 57, 120
Polymorphism, 31, 120
Polypeptide, 96, 102, 120
Polysaccharide, 97, 120
Postmenopausal, 40, 107, 117, 120
Postnatal, 15, 120
Practice Guidelines, 78, 120
Precursor, 97, 99, 105, 106, 120, 126, 127
Predisposition, 68, 120
Premenopausal, 11, 120
Prenatal, 14, 105, 120
Presumptive, 13, 120
Prevalence, 9, 35, 38, 51, 120
Progesterone, 40, 41, 42, 52, 64, 120, 124
Progression, 97, 120
Progressive, 100, 102, 107, 116, 120
Proline, 102, 111, 120
Promoter, 14, 120
Prophase, 13, 117, 120
Prospective study, 114, 121
Prostate, 117, 121
Protein S, 52, 99, 121
Proteolytic, 99, 102, 121
Protocol, 108, 121
Psychic, 114, 115, 121
Puberty, 6, 44, 121
Public Health, 5, 78, 121
Public Policy, 77, 121
Pulmonary, 16, 99, 103, 121
Purines, 121, 123
Pyrimidines, 121, 123

R
Race, 116, 121
Radiation, 107, 113, 121, 122, 128
Radiation therapy, 107, 113, 121, 128
Radioactive, 110, 112, 113, 116, 117, 122, 128
Radiolabeled, 99, 113, 122, 128
Radiotherapy, 99, 113, 122, 128

Randomized, 7, 24, 40, 122
Receptivity, 59, 122
Receptor, 4, 6, 8, 9, 19, 21, 25, 29, 31, 36, 38, 57, 97, 107, 122
Receptors, Steroid, 9, 122
Recombinant, 12, 57, 122, 127
Recombination, 15, 108, 122
Rectum, 97, 108, 112, 121, 122
Refer, 1, 100, 102, 117, 122
Refraction, 122, 124
Regimen, 28, 62, 122
Remission, 54, 122
Reproductive cells, 108, 122
Resorption, 107, 117, 122
Rheology, 118, 122
Risk factor, 23, 30, 50, 53, 121, 122
Rubber, 6, 95, 122

S
Salivary, 123
Salivary glands, 123
Saponins, 123, 124
Screening, 5, 18, 30, 38, 53, 102, 123
Secretion, 39, 40, 56, 95, 101, 104, 109, 111, 112, 113, 114, 116, 123, 126
Segregation, 43, 122, 123
Selective estrogen receptor modulator, 123, 125
Sella Turcica, 119, 123
Semen, 69, 105, 121, 123
Seminiferous tubule, 6, 112, 123, 124
Senescence, 6, 123
Senile, 117, 123
Serine, 8, 123
Serologic, 111, 123
Serum, 21, 25, 32, 36, 52, 53, 59, 69, 96, 102, 109, 116, 123, 127
Sex Characteristics, 96, 117, 121, 123, 125
Sicca, 43, 123
Signs and Symptoms, 26, 122, 123
Skeletal, 7, 96, 123
Skeleton, 123, 124
Skin test, 20, 124
Skull, 124, 125
Small intestine, 110, 113, 124
Soma, 124
Somatic, 6, 10, 13, 42, 70, 106, 116, 124
Somatic cells, 13, 70, 116, 124
Specialist, 84, 124
Species, 13, 110, 116, 121, 124, 125, 126, 127, 128
Specificity, 51, 95, 124
Spectrum, 4, 124

Sperm, 96, 101, 108, 122, 123, 124
Spermatozoa, 123, 124
Sporadic, 30, 68, 124
Steroid, 15, 20, 25, 27, 28, 50, 55, 56, 59, 97, 104, 117, 122, 123, 124
Stimulus, 105, 124
Stomach, 106, 108, 110, 113, 124
Stool, 112, 124
Stress, 7, 118, 120, 123, 124
Stroke, 16, 76, 125
Stroma, 10, 125
Styrene, 123, 125
Subspecies, 124, 125
Substance P, 115, 123, 125
Substrate, 106, 125
Superoxide, 7, 125
Superoxide Dismutase, 7, 125
Supplementation, 61, 125
Suppression, 26, 31, 40, 56, 57, 59, 104, 125
Survival Rate, 7, 125

T
Tamoxifen, 11, 123, 125
Telomere, 32, 125
Temporal, 6, 125
Teratoma, 101, 125
Testicular, 6, 107, 125
Testis, 97, 101, 106, 108, 117, 125
Testosterone, 6, 14, 53, 56, 97, 125
Thorax, 95, 125
Threonine, 8, 123, 125
Thrombosis, 113, 121, 125
Thyroid, 51, 100, 111, 125, 126
Thyroid Gland, 126
Thyroiditis, 54, 126
Thyrotropin, 111, 126
Tissue, 21, 97, 98, 99, 101, 102, 103, 106, 109, 111, 112, 113, 114, 115, 116, 119, 120, 124, 125, 126, 128
Tomography, 99, 126
Toxic, iv, 125, 126
Toxicity, 62, 126
Toxicology, 64, 78, 126
Toxins, 97, 106, 112, 116, 126
Trachea, 115, 125, 126
Transcription Factors, 4, 14, 126
Transdermal, 24, 126

Transfection, 14, 99, 108, 126
Transforming Growth Factor beta, 8, 126
Translating, 14, 126
Translocate, 8, 126
Translocation, 23, 29, 37, 39, 40, 44, 45, 126
Transplantation, 102, 105, 115, 126
Trees, 122, 126
Tremor, 4, 127
Trophic, 10, 127
Tryptophan, 102, 127
Tuberculosis, 114, 127
Tumor Necrosis Factor, 24, 127
Type 2 diabetes, 61, 127

U
Urinary, 112, 127
Urine, 99, 112, 127
Uterine Contraction, 95, 127
Uterus, 95, 101, 104, 106, 115, 118, 120, 127

V
Vagina, 101, 115, 127
Vaginal, 68, 127
Vascular, 105, 112, 118, 119, 126, 127
Vasomotor, 107, 127
Vector, 113, 127
Vein, 117, 127
Vesicular, 109, 127
Veterinary Medicine, 77, 127
Virilism, 111, 127
Virulence, 126, 127
Viruses, 95, 107, 115, 127
Viscera, 124, 127
Vitro, 10, 12, 41, 42, 128
Vivo, 128

W
White blood cell, 97, 114, 116, 119, 128
Windpipe, 125, 128
Wound Healing, 113, 128

X
Xenograft, 97, 128
X-ray, 99, 113, 117, 121, 122, 128
X-ray therapy, 113, 128

Y
Yeasts, 119, 128

Z
Zona Pellucida, 44, 128
Zygote, 103, 116, 128